DYSLEXIA IN CHILDREN:
NEW RESEARCH

Dyslexia in Children: New Research

Christopher B. Hayes
Editor

Nova Science Publishers, Inc.
New York

NOTICE TO THE READER

The Publisher has taken reasonable care in the preparation of this book, but makes no expressed or implied warranty of any kind and assumes no responsibility for any errors or omissions. No liability is assumed for incidental or consequential damages in connection with or arising out of information contained in this book. The Publisher shall not be liable for any special, consequential, or exemplary damages resulting, in whole or in part, from the readers' use of, or reliance upon, this material.

This publication is designed to provide accurate and authoritative information with regard to the subject matter covered herein. It is sold with the clear understanding that the Publisher is not engaged in rendering legal or any other professional services. If legal or any other expert assistance is required, the services of a competent person should be sought. FROM A DECLARATION OF PARTICIPANTS JOINTLY ADOPTED BY A COMMITTEE OF THE AMERICAN BAR ASSOCIATION AND A COMMITTEE OF PUBLISHERS.

LIBRARY OF CONGRESS CATALOGING-IN-PUBLICATION DATA
Dyslexia in children : new research / Christopher B. Hayes, editor.
 p. cm.
Includes index.
ISBN 1-59454-969-9
1. Dyslexia. 2. Communicative disorders in children. 3. Reading disability. I. Hayes, Christopher B.
RJ496.A5D97   2007
618.92'8553--dc22   2005037619

Published by Nova Science Publishers, Inc. ✦New York

CONTENTS

PREFACE

Dyslexia is a brain-based type of learning disability that specifically impairs a person's ability to read. Although the disorder varies from person to person, common characteristics among people with dyslexia are difficulty with phonological processing (the manipulation of sounds) and/or rapid visual-verbal responding. The syndrome of dyslexia does not imply low intelligence or poor educational potential, and is independent of race and social background. Although dyslexia seems to be more prevalent among males than females, the exact ratio is unknown: the most commonly quoted figures are between 3:1 and 5:1. The evidence suggests that in at least two-thirds of cases, dyslexia has a genetic cause, but in some cases birth difficulties may play a role.

Dyslexia may overlap with related conditions such as dyspraxia, attention deficit disorder (with or without hyperactivity) and dysphasia. In childhood, its effects can be mis-attributed to emotional or behavioral disorders. By adulthood, many dyslexics will have developed sophisticated compensating strategies that may mask their difficulties. This new book presents state-of-the-art research in this dynamic field.

A remedial spelling training approach is presented in chapter 1 which systematically combines certain visualizing and verbalizing methods to foster dyslexic students' orthographic knowledge and strategy use. Since children and adolescents with severe spelling difficulties show, for the most part, a considerable lack in knowing and following orthographic rules, educational intervention procedures should facilitate their understanding of those spelling regularities and enable them to master related decision-making steps more successfully. Therefore, the development of orthographic competencies requires systematic instruction methods which can help to clarify the concrete rule meanings and identify the separate rule components – and then, also being effective in initiating and strengthening subsequent strategic spelling routines. For that purpose, the current spelling training approach essentially depends upon an integrative application of algorithmic graphs and verbal self-instructions: it illustrates a certain spelling rule by mapping its components and decision-making criteria as an algorithmic flowchart. A certain spelling problem is to be solved by gradually determining each algorithmic criterion. The students trace their partial results step by step with a colored pencil in an algorithmic flow chart, and instruct themselves by thinking aloud until they can solve the target word spelling. Visualization and verbalization are intended to focus the students' attention, cognitions, and behaviors on the algorithmic rule components for enhancing their task orientation and self-regulation skills. To that degree, the intervention must provide an intensive and consistent cognitive modeling phase as well as a broad range of special training materials which, in particular, are comprised of various algorithmic and self-instructional task formats. When the students become more familiar and proficient with these learning modalities they may then reduce their overt self-instructions and increasingly try to operate in terms of inner speech processing – so that they are finally able to use algorithmic decision-making as an individually well-established and successful spelling strategy. Empirical analyses of treatment outcomes in four training cohorts, including children and adolescents with severe spelling disabilities, could demonstrate statistically significant gains in the students' spelling test performances. The training was administered in single-case or small group sessions and took about 80 hours on an average. In each cohort, the differences between pre- and post-test data were more than 10 T-score points and reached a reasonably strong effect size (d > 2). The students' advances could be proved in both systematically trained and, to a somewhat lesser degree, only incidentally considered spelling areas. In comparison, in spelling areas being left untrained up to the post-test measures, the students' gains in performance appeared to be smaller and less clear. Furthermore, data revealed evidence for the remedial effects largely to reach the same magnitude across different teaching persons. In another study, the achievement-related pre- and post-test measures from an experimental group and a control group, both including students with severe spelling disabilities, were compared. The treatment was administered in single-case sessions and took about 34 hours. Post-test results could demonstrate statistically significant advantages in the experimental students' spelling test performances. Overall, they showed better spelling results in systematically trained spelling areas, compared to only incidentally considered or even untrained spelling areas. Taken altogether, these preliminary findings are likely to support the systematic use of visualizing and verbalizing methods in remedial spelling training and should encourage further evaluation efforts.

Dyslexic children are characterized by a phoneme awareness deficit and the associated problems in performing decoding. In particular, most reading errors are due to confusions between phonemes which differ on minimal traits (especially voiced-unvoiced oppositions). Dyslexics may have a poorer categorical perception of certain contrasts. In chapter 2, the authors hypothesize that specific audio-visual training which aids phonetic feature perception could help dyslexic children to specify phonemic representations. Consequently, they should not confuse close phonemes on the phonetic features which could facilitate written word processing. The aim was to test the effectiveness of an audio-visual training program designed to improve the discrimination of the phonetic feature of voicing on dyslexic children's recognition of written words. Sixteen dyslexic children were separated into two equal groups strictly matched on educational and cognitive levels, as well as on reading level which was assessed using a standardized word reading test. The children in the experimental group received the audio-visual training whereas the children in the control group used a computerized "talking book" program. This system program enabled the children to read sentences on the computer under whole word and syllable feedback conditions. The reading material consisted of a set of stories selected from children's literature. The experimental training focused on paired-item voicing oppositions and involved six pairs of phonemes: /p/-/b/; /t/-/d/; /k/-/g/; /f/-/v/; /s/-/z/ and /ch/-/j/. A traditional pre-test, interventiontraining phase, and post-test design was used. Tests included a word recognition test and reading comprehension were tested. The results show the impact of audio-visual training on the performances of the dyslexic children in the word reading task. It proved possible to improve phonological representations by means of training which involved both phonological and orthographic units. The effectiveness of this audio-visual training is discussed both in the light of the phonetic model - the phonological deficits in dyslexic children may be partly due to impairments in the phonetic organization of phoneme detectors, as well as in terms of a connectionist model of reading development.

Developmental dyslexia has been associated with an auditory rate processing deficit as part of a cross-modal temporal dysfunction. The empirical evidence for the co-occurrence of visual and auditory impairments is not conclusive, however. One possibility is that the discordant findings are moderated by the subject's age. In chapter 3, the authors investigate cross-sectionally whether a visual temporal deficit in children with dyslexia disappears through development. The same experimental tasks as used in an earlier study involving 13-year-olds were administered to 11 year-old dyslexic and normally literate children. Auditory rate processing was assessed by means of a syllable-discrimination task; visual processing was indexed by judgments of temporal order of lightness changes. As a main result, dyslexic children exhibited higher visual thresholds than the controls did. This was in contrast to what was observed in older participants. Auditory data of young and older dyslexic children yielded two subgroups: one benefiting from temporal extension of stop consonant-vowel syllables and the other showing a balanced performance profile across consonant durations. Both younger dyslexics and older controls demonstrated no relationship between auditory accuracy and visual thresholds. In contrast, significant relationships were found in the younger control and older dyslexic group. The findings suggest the co-occurrence of visual and auditory impairments in young children with dyslexia. Visual processing deficits, however, seem to ameliorate across development. Hence, younger dyslexic children may have deficits in both modalities, but older dyslexics may not show co-occurrence of visual and auditory impairments.

Some evidence associates dyslexia, both developmental and acquired, with binocular instability, reduced amplitude of accomodation and reduced contrast sensitivity for both low spatial frequencies and uniform field flicker as described in chapter 4. If vision plays a dominant role in the guidance of movements, cerebellar lesions produce profound deficits in visuomotor control, considering that visual information is integrated in lobule VIc and VII of the caudal vermis important for the control of both smooth pursuit and target-directed saccades. Considering these perspectives, the authors studied 5 young patients with selective vermian/paravermian lesions, and 5 young adults with selective hemispheric cerebellar lesion, who before did never complain reading troubles, in order to detect eventual difficulties or abnormalities in reading process. They have compared the results to those obtained by a group of normal volunteers. They suggest that only vermian patients (and not those with hemispheric lesions) respond imperfectly to normal controlling influences exerted by the vermis region on the SC and the pontine nuclei; therefore, this may cause inappropriate eye positioning sufficient to decrease the ability of reading. In particular, they hypothesize that vermian lesions produce a defective control of saccadic movements, fundamental for the execution of the reading task.

Deficits in auditory or visual perception or in saccade control contribute to problems in acquiring reading and spelling. The corresponding examination of the perceptual and optomotor skills have shown developmental deficits in comparison with age matched control groups. Chapter 5 describes the development, deficits, and training effects of a special visual function called subitizing. This function enables subjects to recognize immediately (= subito, lat.) a small number of items even when they were presented only for short periods of time.

In chapter 6 different fields of dyslexia research will be analysed in the view of Lakatos "research programmes". The aim is two-folded; to try and see if his intended meaning of "research programmes" is applicable to dyslexia research; and to use his philosophy of science to gain a meta-view, and hence better insight into the current status of dyslexia research. The high frequency of dyslexia in the population, its educational implications, and its many intertwining scientific and clinical aspects, invite for a useful framework to organise the knowledge.

One hypothesis about the aetiology of developmental dyslexia is that it is partially caused by a deficit of the magnocellular pathway. Previous research has indicated that the magnocellular system is in fact involved in the identification of flanked letters, the basic building blocks of text. Importantly, people with developmental dyslexia have indeed been found to experience problems with identifying flanked letters. Therefore, in chapter 7, it was tested directly whether the dyslexic problems with flanked-letter identification are due to a magnocellular deficit. The authors did this by comparing the single- and the flanked-letter-identification ability of university students with ($N = 24$) and without ($N = 24$) developmental dyslexia using pure colour contrast and pure luminance contrast between characters and background. The contrast manipulation can be considered a manipulation of magnocellular activity since the magnocellular system is relatively more sensitive to luminance modulation than is the parvocellular system, whereas the latter is the more sensitive to colour variation. In line with expectations, the dyslexic participants had difficulty identifying flanked letters and they also performed poorly in a coherent-motion task, presumably reflecting poor magnocellular function. The contrast manipulation, however, failed to differentiate between the two groups. Possible explanations for these apparently discrepant findings are discussed.

Recent studies have shown the critical role of the ability to actively select visual information (attentional focusing) in developmental dyslexia. A program specifically devised by Geiger and Lettvin to train selection of visual information and small-scale focusing has been tried out with a group of 16 dyslexic children as reported in chapter 8. The results after a three-months training have been compared with those obtained by another group of 11 dyslexic children after the same period of customary reading training in a speech-therapy context. All children were assessed on reading, spelling and phonemic awareness and their FRFs (Form-Resolving Fields), i.e. the extent of their field of correct visual recognition, were measured. The children who followed the experimental training improved their reading and spelling performances as much as the children who were treated by speech therapists (no significant differences were observed between the two groups). However, separate analyses reveal that improvements after treatment for the experimental group on reading accuracy, reading speed, spelling, phonemic awareness reached statistical significance. The group receiving customary speech therapy, on the other hand, shows significant improvements on spelling only.

In: Dyslexia in Children: New Research
Editor: Christopher B. Hayes, pp. 1-45

ISBN 1-59454-969-9

Chapter 1

THE SYSTEMATIC USE OF VISUALIZING AND VERBALIZING METHODS IN REMEDIAL SPELLING TRAINING: CONCEPTUAL ISSUES, PRACTICAL APPLICATIONS, AND EMPIRICAL FINDINGS

Günter Faber
Arbeitsstelle für pädagogische Entwicklung und Förderung Goslar (Germany)

ABSTRACT

A remedial spelling training approach is presented which systematically combines certain visualizing and verbalizing methods to foster dyslexic students' orthographic knowledge and strategy use. Since children and adolescents with severe spelling difficulties show, for the most part, a considerable lack in knowing and following orthographic rules, educational intervention procedures should facilitate their understanding of those spelling regularities and enable them to master related decision-making steps more successfully. Therefore, the development of orthographic competencies requires systematic instruction methods which can help to clarify the concrete rule meanings and identify the separate rule components – and then, also being effective in initiating and strengthening subsequent strategic spelling routines. For that purpose, the current spelling training approach essentially depends upon an integrative application of algorithmic graphs and verbal self-instructions: it illustrates a certain spelling rule by mapping its components and decision-making criteria as an algorithmic flowchart. A certain spelling problem is to be solved by gradually determining each algorithmic criterion. The students trace their partial results step by step with a colored pencil in an algorithmic flow chart, and instruct themselves by thinking aloud until they can solve the target word spelling. Visualization and verbalization are intended to focus the students' attention, cognitions, and behaviors on the algorithmic rule components for enhancing their task orientation and self-regulation skills. To that degree, the intervention must provide an intensive and consistent cognitive modeling phase as well as a broad range of special training materials which, in particular, are comprised of various algorithmic and self-instructional task formats. When the students become more familiar and proficient with these learning modalities they may then reduce their overt self-instructions and increasingly try to operate in terms of inner speech processing – so that they are finally able to use algorithmic decision-making as an individually well-established and successful spelling strategy. Empirical analyses of treatment outcomes in four training cohorts, including children and adolescents with severe spelling disabilities, could demonstrate statistically significant gains in the students' spelling test performances. The training was administered in single-case or small group sessions and took about 80 hours on an average. In each cohort, the differences between pre- and post-test data were more than 10 T-score points and reached a reasonably strong effect size (d > 2). The students' advances could be proved in both systematically trained and, to a somewhat lesser degree, only incidentally considered spelling areas. In comparison, in spelling areas being left untrained up to the post-test measures, the students' gains in performance appeared to be smaller and less clear. Furthermore, data revealed evidence for the remedial effects largely to reach the same magnitude across different teaching persons. In another study, the achievement-related pre- and post-test measures from an experimental group and a control group, both including students with severe spelling disabilities, were compared. The treatment was administered in single-case sessions and took about 34 hours. Post-test results could demonstrate statistically significant advantages in the experimental students' spelling test performances. Overall, they showed better spelling results in systematically trained spelling areas, compared to only incidentally considered or even untrained spelling areas. Taken altogether, these preliminary findings are likely to support the systematic use of visualizing and verbalizing methods in remedial spelling training and should encourage further evaluation efforts.

CONCEPTUAL ISSUES

Beyond the Mastering of Phonological Spelling Skills: Orthographic Knowledge and Strategy Problems in Dyslexic Students

With the help of mostly long-term and intensive remedial training, many dyslexic students are enabled to significantly achieve improved phonological spelling skills, reducing their relevant error ratio at the same time. However, their problems in applying orthographical rules tend to persist and increase at higher grade levels (Klicpera and Schabmann, 1993): as such, many of the students concerned have no or only scarce knowledge of the important orthographic rules and are not familiar with their implications – and thus they do not follow structurally adequate criteria as much as those seeming subjectively plausible to them. Often they resort to their existing phonological spelling skills, and they try in vain to master the critical word items in terms of phonological correctness (Bailet, 1990; Carlisle, 1987; Darch, Kim, Johnson and James, 2000; Frith, 1985; Manis and Morrison, 1985; Steffler, 2004). Due to their errors, these students then seem irritated and disappointed over their unsuccessful spelling efforts as they have, from their viewpoint, genuinely pondered over the words and could even come up with an explanation for their decision to choose the spelling they used. In addition however, there are also those students who, on the one hand, are formally familiar with the rules required, and who are able to recite the orthographically correct reasons for the spelling of certain word items – who are, on the other hand however, partially or completely lacking effective approaches to a successful application of their knowledge. These students are then unable to apply their knowledge of orthographic rules in a consistent, certain, and swift way as they do not or only fragmentarily engage in relevant considerations. Due to the pressures in terms of time and demands they experience in the dictation situation they often tend to give up and resort to intuitive guessing to a large extent.

In light of their cumulated failure experiences, the students concerned are gradually arriving at the conclusion that spelling and writing with orientation to orthographic regularities is not really helpful to them, and that the rules conveyed to them in class do not offer reliable solutions, according to their experience, to significantly reduce their own error ratio. Over time however, and as a result of the above, there is an increased risk that they are hardly able any longer to recognize clues and leads so as to master their individual difficulties. This in turn may result in motivational orientations characterized by resignation, helplessness, and avoidance, the foreseeable effects of which, in terms of missing learning success, are contributing to a further stabilization of the existing problem situation (Carroll, Maughan, Goodman and Meltzer, 2005; Faber, 2000, Faber, 2002d,e; Heiervang, Stevenson, Lund and Hugdahl, 2001; Humphrey and Mullins, 2002; Licht and Kistner, 1986; Nolen-Hoeksema, Girgus and Seligman, 1986; Poskiparta, Niemi, Lepola, Ahtola and Laine, 2003; Sideridis, 2003; Tobias, 1992).

Enhancing Dyslexic Students' Orthographic Competencies: Some Methodical Considerations and Instructional Guidelines

Therefore, the task in remedial spelling training is to enhance, round off, or catch up on the orthographic skills of the students concerned, the acquirement of which had been unsuccessful for them so far – so as to avoid, last but not least, the motivational and socio-emotional long-term effects of failure experiences accumulated in the individual (Betz and Breuninger, 1993; Cohen, 1986; Humphrey, 2003). The development and persistence of these learning difficulties can be traced back essentially to fundamental knowledge and strategy deficiencies: the students concerned are lacking relevant knowledge with regard to the critical demands; in addition, they do not possess suitable metacognitive planning and control concepts for the acquirement of appropriate learning strategies – or they are unable to adequately apply solution approaches formally known to them. Therefore, adequate remedial interventions have to teach students the knowledge of relevant rules in an understandable way, and useful behavioral patterns with regard to the instruction strategy have to be worked out so as to bring this knowledge to application (Baird and White, 1982; Larkin and Ellis, 2004; Mannhaupt, 1999; Reid, 1988).

In particular, learning theories from the view of action psychology point up the necessity of an instructional approach which enables the students to understand the underlying logic of a certain spelling rule and to form a cognitive concept or tool for further problem solving in that given spelling domain (Arievitch and Stetsenko, 2000; Gal'perin, 1989a,b,c). In this sense, the training must include systematic orientation guides for the presentation of the object of learning in a way suitable to the students, as well as effective structuring remedies for a proper acquirement of the skills on the part of the students. Accordingly, the task of gradually developing relevant skills requires, first of all, finding suitable ways of conveying orthographic rules which guarantee that the issues at hand can actually be followed and understood by the students. Most of all, this requires considerations in the direction of resolving the verbal, abstract complexity of orthographic rules by subdividing them into single information chunks of a concrete nature which, when looking at them from the students´ view, seem logically consistent, reliable, and mentally controllable. To that degree, an orientation basis significantly enhancing the learning process can be achieved by implementing visualization and verbalization methods subdividing the orthographic regulations into their characteristic sub-operations, thus presenting them in a methodical sequence of relevant decision criteria – in symbolic-graphic form and as descriptive as possible (Clarke, 1991). In this way, the students receive materialized, quasi prototypic patterns of thought/action which are supposed to enable them to acquire knowledge and certainty of the relevant rules in clearly structured steps. If these conditions are fulfilled the next task is to implement adequate strategies making it possible for the students to carry over their acquired knowledge of the orthographic rules to corresponding spelling routines, and to apply it autonomously in order to meet orthographic demands. Therefore, the orthographic remedial approach has to be relocated from the physical activity level into the consciousness of the students, habitualizing it there as a behaviorally active pattern of thinking. Thus, the acquirement of skills and strategies is supposed to take place by educationally initiated and monitored internalization processes. In order to achieve this, it is absolutely essential, in the view of action psychology, to carry over the action from the exterior to the interior speech by putting the orthographic rule processing completely into language (Bodrova and Leong, 1998; Galperin, 1989a), having the students commenting their rule application aloud – until they master it so well that they gradually need less and less time for the operation and are finally able to do without verbal teacher assistance. Now the students approach the orthographic solution without materialized structuring or overt self-instructions, and they have successfully automatized it as a continuous spelling strategy.

Overall, these considerations result in important methodical clues and leads for a systematic remedial training of the students' orthographic skills (Figure 1): the successful acquirement and application of orthographic rules may be facilitated significantly if one can successfully manage to subdivide the complex meaning of the rules into clearly structured intermediate algorithmic steps which can easily be visualized – and if one can also successfully manage to support the acquirement of these intermediate algorithmic steps with consistent verbalizing methods. In doing so, the acquirement of orthographic spelling skills may predominantly dependent upon the implementation of suitable visualizing methods, the development of relevant solution strategies, and most of all, the use of suitable verbalizing methods. This in turn does not necessarily have to mean that the acquirement of skills and the development of solution strategies in physical action should be considered apart from each other. Much rather, it may be crucial for the success of the remedial process to be able to combine both instruction approaches (and thus the implementation of visualizing and verbalizing methods as well) as closely as possible.

For the beginning stages of the translating experience of the intermediate algorithmic steps into language and their subsequent consolidation with regard to the learning strategy, it seems methodically self-evident to utilize and adjust the principles of cognitive modeling and self-instructional learning (Meichenbaum and Asarnow, 1979) – as their efficiency in the development of strategic skills on the part of the students has been proven sufficiently long since, across a wide range of educational problems and school grades (Ellis, Deshler, Lens, Schumaker and Clark, 1991; Harris, 1990; Miller and Brewster, 1992; Montague, 1997; Schunk, 1986).

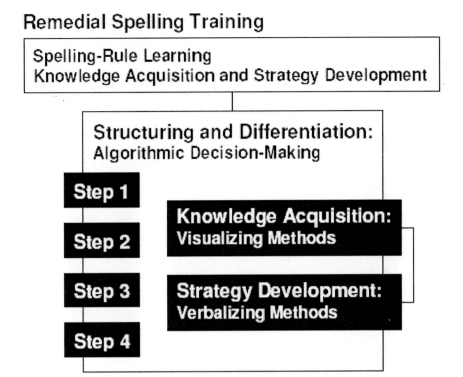

Figure 1. Knowledge acquisition and strategy development in remedial spelling training: The crucial role of visualizing and verbalizing methods.

Visualizing and Verbalizing Methods in Existing Training Programmes: A Brief Overview and Discussion

In more or less close alignment with these conceptual issues, various training concepts exist in the meantime that aim at the systematic development of orthographic skills and strategies. Their performance-enhancing effects have been empirically proven, at least in part, as well (Mannhaupt, 2003; Scheerer-Neumann, 1993).

As such, different approaches attempt to teach the students selected orthographic rules by using algorithmic plans, and by providing a reliable sequence of concrete mental steps to facilitate students' learning of orthographic spelling rules. Occasionally, these algorithms are imparted to the students as short formulas or self-instructional phrases, but the majority consists of graphical solutions. With the aid of relevant cue cards or flow charts, the students are encouraged to implement pattern and procedure of the rule, thus being able to arrive at the orthographically correct way of spelling and writing by themselves (Kossow, 1979; Lechner, 1985; Mann, 1991; Matthes, 1994; Röber-Siekmeyer, 1993; Scheerer-Neumann, 1988; Schulte-Körne and Mathwig, 2001; Stolla, 2000; Tijms and Hoeks, 2005).

As of now, there are only relatively few programmes that include procedures with the objective of helping the students internalize the algorithmic steps pertaining to an orthographic rule learned by them, by means of verbal self-instruction, and to carry over these skills to relevant action strategies. One step in this direction is the technique of verbally commenting the consecutive steps of writing. With the help of self-instructional steps voiced aloud, the students are supposed to focus their attention on word parts prone to orthographic error and apply their skills acquired (Weigt, 1994). Other programmes have resorted more to the method of cognitive modeling and adjusted it accordingly. They subdivide the orthographic steps towards the solution in clearly structured behavioral sequences which, at first, are presented to the students by a person modeling the skill application thinking aloud. Then the students take over these self-instructions. By consistently practicing the single action steps and self-instructional approaches, the students are supposed to successively develop the behavior aimed at and required for the solution, eventually being able to automatize it as an orthographic strategy. However, the relevant programmes have been tested in the framework of pertinent research projects exclusively, and only a few orthographic rules have been taken into consideration by them. As such, findings with regard to a strategic coverage of a comprehensive repertoire of orthographic rules by means of verbal self-instruction are still outstanding (Mäki, Vauras and Vainio, 2002; Nock, Sikorski and Thiel, 1988; Scheerer-Neumann, 1979; Walter, Bigga and Bischof, 1995).

Undoubtedly, the various programmes show interesting possibilities with regard to graphic algorithms and verbal self-instruction approaches for the development of students' orthographic skills – but at the same time, a conceptual development potential is recognizable: as measured by pertinent concepts in action psychology, the algorithms used turn out to be quite complex illustrations of orthographic solution methods. It seems that they are less suitable as a learning tool for the acquirement of the problem-solving skill, and that they serve more as a recollection aid for the utilization of orthographic skills already acquired by the individual. In addition, the self-instruction approaches employed operationalize the specific problem-solving behavior, as regards content, still relatively inaccurately – for instance, when they do not reflect the sequence of the relevant orthographic action in sufficient detail, and when the wording does not mirror the specific rules adequately (Thackwray, Meyers, Schleser and Cohen, 1985). And finally, most programmes focus either on the use of algorithmic problem-solving plans or on the application of self-instructive modeling techniques. In contrast, the possibilities of a closer combination of both aspects, originally envisioned in action psychology as well (Gal'perin, 1989a), seem hardly utilized. In this sense, training approaches with a more method-integrating character can make a significant contribution to the continuative structuring and individualization of the remedial training of dyslexic students.

Visualizing and Verbalizing Orthographic Learning Complexities: A Remedial Spelling Training Approach

As a consequence of the conceptual limitations of the existing programmes, there is a need to further develop the approach to a systematic enhancement of students' orthographic skills in two respects (Faber, 2001a, 2002c, 2003c):

- In the phase of initial exploration and gradual acquirement of orthographic rules, the spelling training should already utilize algorithmic problem-solving plans which guarantee a clear, descriptive, and distinct illustration of the relevant rule meaning –

requiring for its use only relatively little previous knowledge on the part of the students. The work with methods of this kind could contribute to a more targeted initiation and organization of the orthographic learning process.

- For the purpose of a successive development of orthographic learning strategies, the spelling training should, from the start, directly combine verbal self-instruction methods with the application of visualized problem-solving algorithms so that the significant algorithmic decision steps can be practiced by the students by memorizing them aloud with the aim that they can be implemented later on without visualizing and verbalizing methods. This combination of algorithmic problem-solving plans and verbal self-instructions could orient the strategically necessary transition from exterior and interior speaking closer to the relevant orthographic skills – and thus significantly facilitate the initiation and habitualization of orthographic learning strategies from the beginning.

In this sense, remedial spelling training aims at a systematic combination of conveying orthographic rule knowledge and developing rule-specific strategy use, as well as bundling both learning aspects in such a way that they have a synergetic effect upon each other, and that they can be optimized with regard to their efficiency.

From a methodical viewpoint, this requires in particular an algorithmic problem-solving plan which is capable of both structuring the acquirement of orthographic knowledge and facilitating the development of orthographic strategies simultaneously – by providing the specific problem-solving steps as well as the self-instruction steps at the same time. In this regard, an algorithmic flow chart (Figure 2) has proven to be a suitable method

- that focuses the students' attention on the target word, first of all, introducing a reflexive problem-solving action,
- that determines the relevant orthographic problem as a concrete issue in question,
- that introduces an algorithmically structured problem-solving approach to clear the issue in question with definite decision criteria in clearly structured intermediate steps,
- that presents the algorithmically founded spelling of the target word as a reliable solution,
- and that eventually carries over this solution to an orthographically adequate spelling of the target word.

The application of this problem-solving plan has to be demonstrated by the teacher first by thinking aloud. In the course of this, the teacher also informs the students in detail of the meaning of the problem-solving algorithm and the benefits of the thinking aloud technique for one's own enhancement of orthographic skills (Pressley, 1986; Schunk and Rice, 1987). Under these circumstances, the students can test and practice the problem-solving plan with the teacher's guidance. At first, they apply the plan by thinking aloud, without exception. In doing so, they follow the algorithmic plan determined by them on a respective worksheet step by step with a colored pencil. In the case of errors or uncertainties, the teacher discontinues the ongoing solution attempt and starts to determine the correct solution approach together with the students, repetitively modeling the correct step if needed. In this way, each target word is analyzed by itself before a decision is made. Both the self-instructions and the colored marking of the solution approach should contribute to the students slowing down in their solution behavior, thus replacing impulsive guessing with reflexive action patterns. At the same time, they should be able to perceive their proceeding more consciously and control it more precisely, as the combination of visualized algorithms and verbal self-instruction renders the own success/failure experience more comprehensible. The flowchart helps to precisely locate and promptly eliminate any difficulties in executing a certain problem-solving step.

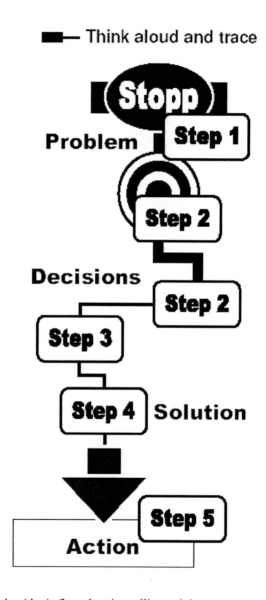

Figure 2. Principle of an algorithmic flow chart in spelling training

For the systematic work with algorithmic flow charts of this nature, methodically adequate practice materials in particular play a central role. They have to depict the orthographic demands using algorithmically formatted exercise types consistently enabling the students to convert the orthographic skills acquired by them into a strategically adequate behavior (Faber, 2002c, 2003c, 2005c).

PRACTICAL APPLICATIONS

Algorithmic and Self-Instructional Task Formats

For the systematic acquirement of orthographic skills and the development of pertinent learning strategies it is necessary to have a wide range of suitable materials at one's disposal. They should be formatted in such a way that they illustrate the principle of the problem-solving algorithm leading to an application of the relevant orthographic rule with confidence by using graphic illustrations and strategically structured handling steps. When working on these tasks, the students should be able to realize at any time what the single problem-solving steps are, and in what sequence they have to be applied. At the same time, these types of tasks should always optionally combine working on the critical word material and verbalizing self-instructive comments with regard to the spelling strategy, providing proper assistance for that purpose – so that the mental consolidation of the individual's knowledge of the solution approach is already purposefully supported by the task structure, according to the student's level of skill, facilitating habitualization of pertinent action routines. When the students are sufficiently certain the relevant problem-solving steps can be abridged and eventually omitted altogether – yet, when difficulties arise they can be reemployed in their entirety. Below, the possibilities of a practical implementation of this principle will be introduced and elucidated, with selected task formats as examples.

Algorithmic Problem-Solving Plans

The algorithmic problem-solving plans illustrate the application of an orthographic rule as a reliable sequence of the single problem-solving steps. In German orthography for example, the consonant g is pronounced as k in numerous nouns, verbs, and adjectives (likewise d as t and b as p). Therefore, only a phonologically correct spelling of these word parts is bound to fail. Accordingly, the students have to master the rule of determining the orthographically correct spelling by establishing the respective basic form and/or plural form. This solution approach is explained to them with the relevant flow chart and its algorithmic sequence of problem-solving steps (Figure 3). The complete application of the algorithm is then demonstrated by thinking aloud, and systematically practiced in combination with the corresponding self-instruction steps. For this purpose, the students take over the decision steps modeled by the teacher, again by thinking aloud, and they follow the solution approach found in each case with a colored pencil on the algorithmic flow chart. The application of this problem-solving plan can be substantiated according to the following pattern: (1) The student is told the word, and he determines the critical word part he/she is supposed to resolve. (2) By thinking aloud, he establishes the basic form of the verb, and (3) he pronounces its two syllables slowly and clearly. In between the syllables he pauses notedly. (4) By thinking aloud, he determines the spoken letter sound, and (5) he decides how to spell and write that word part. (6) Finally, he writes the word with the solution he arrived at into the corresponding box. When the student is sufficiently certain the self-instruction steps thought aloud can be abbreviated, and eventually be omitted altogether. All the student does then is to point at the single problem-solving steps, or he autonomously draws the solution approach on the worksheet. If uncertainties or errors occur, he returns to applying the plan by thinking aloud again. Algorithmic flow charts of this nature exist for all important rules of German orthography (Faber, 2001b, 2002a, 2003a, 2004d).

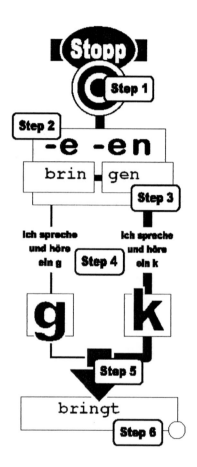

Figure 3. Algorithmic flow chart in the spelling skill area gk (concerning the spelling of explosive consonant sounds)

Algorithmic and Self-Instructive Task Formats

For the purpose of habitualizing this solution approach, with the consolidation of orthographic skills acquired in mind, analogously formatted practice materials with blanks to be filled in are used. They provide appropriately structured solution approaches which are graphically integrated into the task (Figure 4). Working on these tasks involves four steps: (1) The students either find the relevant word by themselves, or they are being told it. They repeat it aloud. (2) By using the decision-making symbols provided in the word box (e.g. for establishing the plural form, or determining vowel length) they clarify the critical word part, and (3) they determine the correct spelling. (4) Finally, they write the word into the corresponding box. First however, the use of this task format has to be modeled by the teacher and practiced with the students step by step. According to the individual level of skill, the decision-making symbols in the second step can be applied by the students, either thinking them aloud, or already silently by means of inner speech processing. In the further course of the exercises, they are gradually fading out, and on the corresponding worksheets they are merely indicated by empty forms to be verbalized, marked, and filled in by the students if required. With further routine acquired, the students should be able to use these algorithmic comprehension aids more and more in a self-instructive manner (Faber, 2002b, 2004d, 2005a,c).

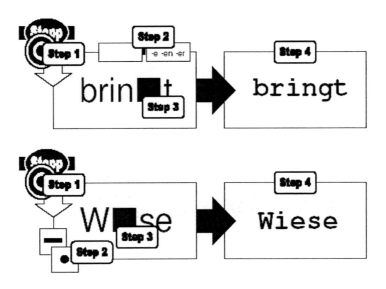

Figure 4. Algorithmic and self-instructional task format: An example

Analysis of Vowel Length

For a number of German orthographic rules it is important to accurately determine the length of the radical vowel – for example, the long i is written as ie, and after a long vowel there is no doubling of consonants (Landerl, 2003). Some students have a very hard time to correctly recognize and pronounce the length of the radical vowel in a word. In such cases, this competency should be developed, controlled, and consolidated systematically. The task format for analyzing vowel length is designed for that purpose (Figure 5); the vowel, pronounced long vs. short, can be "tracked" – spoken out loud – on the graphic template with a pencil, and can be analyzed subsequently. At the beginning it should be thoroughly clarified with the students to what extent they are able, on the one hand, to clearly distinguish vowels with long pronunciation from those with short pronunciation, and on the other hand, to consciously vary the vocal length in the respective word. For this purpose, it has proven helpful to pronounce selected words in a contrasting comparison, first with a long and then with a short vowel – and only then have the students decide which alternative applies. In four consecutive steps, (1) the students are being told a word in normal pronunciation, after which the students pronounce it with both a long and a short vowel. On the worksheet (2) they accompany the long articulation with a line [—] drawn simultaneously, (3) the short articulation with a period [.] placed simultaneously. In case of uncertainties, this procedure should be repeated. Only after a contrasting comparison of the two alternatives (4) do they arrive at a decision. The teacher has to systematically train and practice this procedure with the students. Accompanying the articulations with a respective line or period helps the students to control the deliberately long vs. short pronunciation of a vowel depending upon speech and motion – which in turn enables them to receive a more precise feedback with regard to the articulation realized by them. With more certainty gained, the vowel length spoken can be accompanied and assisted with analogous hand signals by having the students "draw" a clear line in the air with their index finger in the case of long vowels, and having them "place" a period in the air in the case of short ones. However, if it turns out that students have difficulties in mastering certain words with regard to their vowel length, the graphic practice template should always be used again in a targeted manner (Faber, 2004a,d, 2005c).

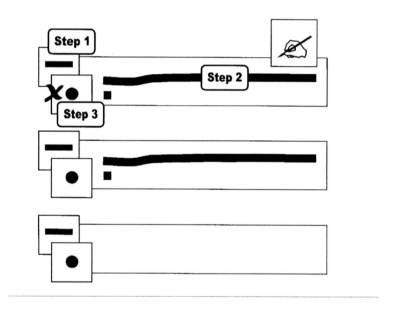

Figure 5. Analysis of vowel length: Visualized and self-instructional task format

Task Formats for Syllable Segmentation

For an adequate implementation of many German orthographic rules, a firm segmentation of words into syllables is indispensable. If students show fundamental difficulties syllablizing the critical word (or its derived or extended form, for that matter), the training should include practice phases pertaining to that particular difficulty. For that purpose, appropriate task formats can be used. They are supposed to slow down the process of syllable segmenting in a targeted manner and help to systematically consolidate them in different ways. An important aspect with all syllable exercises is the deceleration, the strict observance of pausing in between any two syllables. This is the only way to achieve a conscious speech process with regard to articulation and motorics – so that the students can explore, determine, and utilize their own articulation and phonation when syllablizing a word. The task formats at hand are arranged in such a way that any two-syllable word can be worked on with them – and that the students' syllablzation skills can be developed gradually, and increasingly habitualized subsequently. In the respective training process they should, by all means, be used on a regular basis, but each time only within a brief work phase. As such, one task format (Figure 6) combines the syllable segmentation of a target word with the generation of the frequently difficult initial sound of consonant accumulations (inter alia br, dr, gl, gr, kl, kn, kr, pr, tr) and of critical phoneme-grapheme-relations (sch, sp, st, qu). In doing so, student is being told the word, then he (1) generates the initial sound, determines its spelling, and enters the corresponding letters into the speech bubble. He adopts this solution for the first syllable, then (2) he writes the initial sound into the first syllable box and now starts to articulate this first syllable, (3) the spelling of which he then completes in the box. Finally, (4) he generates the second syllable and enters it into the second syllable box. In all intermediate steps, the student should be enabled, with appropriate assistance and repetitions, to explore and consciously reconstruct the significant articulation and phonation processes by himself. In this regard, the teacher plays a crucial role as a behavioral model (Faber, 2004d).

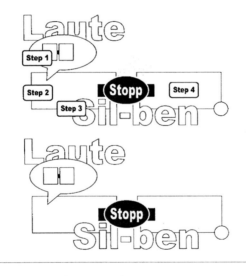

Figure 6. Task format combining the syllable segmentation of a target word with the generation of the frequently difficult initial sound of consonant accumulations

Dictation Formats for Self-Instructive Spelling

For the purpose of systematically practicing self-instructive spelling, dictation formats can be employed which are structured accordingly. They contain various graphic cues aiming at reminding the student of the mental problem-solving approach prior to and increasingly during the writing act as well. The interconnection of thinking and spelling process intended in each case has to be trained first by thinking aloud; when the student is visibly gaining certainty it should be realized silently more and more. For advanced students it should suffice to reconstruct and resolve possible uncertainties or errors in the final verification of results by thinking aloud. Aside from six single word dictations, the format also provides for the spelling of a short sentence (Figure 7). In this way, the transfer of rule-specific spelling skills, controlled by self-instruction, from the limited word level to the orthographically more complex sentence level is supposed to be initiated and consolidated gradually. Optionally, the single word dictations may already take into consideration words from the corresponding sentence. It is of crucial importance here as well that the student reflects on his solution proposal, verbalizing it prior to writing. If needed, the sentence finally to be dictated is repeated any number of times so that the student has sufficient opportunities to analyze and resolve the single words in detail with regard to orthographically critical points: "I try to spell the basic form... in syllables, pausing in between..." When verifying the result, every word spelled correctly is marked accordingly in the corresponding circle. Errors are analyzed together, and various possibilities to avoid these are discussed: "How does the `i´ sound in this word? Pronounce the word again, once short and once long…" (Faber, 2004d).

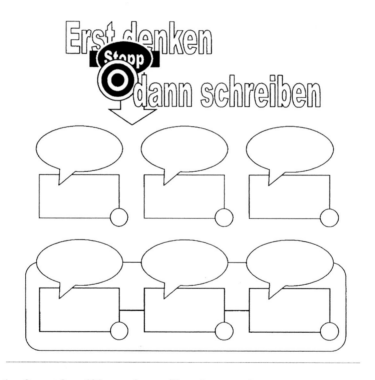

Figure 7. Dictation format for self-instructive spelling: An example

Use of the Materials in Remedial Training

With the systematic use of the algorithmically formatted self-instructive materials, far-reaching possibilities for the enhancement of students' orthographic competencies can be opened up. With regard to their arrangement and application, they offer sufficient opportunities to develop a mode of acquirement geared to the learning requirements of each single student, thus guaranteeing a maximum degree of structured, transparent, and individualized learning (Larkin and Ellis, 2004) – e.g. by targeted variation of the number and complexity of single problem-solving steps, as well as by introduction of alternative concepts and self-instruction approaches. Accordingly, its application seems basically suitable for the training of single individuals and small groups of dyslexic students and adolescents of all levels of education. Both the self-instructions thought aloud and the colored marking of the solution approach on the flowchart should help students, particularly those with attention deficit problems in their problem-solving behavior, to orient it more closely to the task at hand, and to organize it in a more reflexive manner overall (Barkley, 1998; Reid, Trout and Schartz, 2005). Moreover, the graphic problem-solving algorithms can assist the students not only in objectively evolving and rendering comprehensible the respective orthographic rule, but they also provide immediate, action-related feedback with regard to the course and result of their problem-solving approach – which should also contribute to a development of cognitive-motivationally beneficial convictions, as to control and competencies, on a long-term basis. In this regard, it thus seems advantageous when teacher feedback point out expressly method- or strategy related performance attributions, and when these comments mirror the proper mastery in case the students are successful, and vice versa, the lack of adherence to the algorithmic problem-solving steps in case of failures (Clifford, 1990; Tabassam and Grainger, 2003). Finally, the use of the algorithmically formatted self-instructive materials should also be diagnostically helpful by making it possible to provide teachers and students with sufficient information, closely oriented to the actual spelling demands and instructional processes, for a cooperative analysis, planning, and control of the ongoing training situation (Faber, 2003a).

In the meantime, the practical longtime experiences with this approach have led to various supplements and advancements: as of now, algorithmically formatted self-instructive materials for the training of phonological and alphabetical skills exist as well which can serve to support the strategic learning of selected critical phoneme-grapheme-correspondences (Figure 8). In addition, it has turned out that the systematic application of these materials can be combined favorably with other training methods (Topping, 1995; Zutell, 1996).

However, the ways and means of how to implement a systematic spelling training with these materials in the actual training situation always depends upon the concrete student competencies and the teacher – in any case, the materials introduced should provide for sufficient leeway with regard to an individually tailored application (Bodrova and Leong, 1998). Undoubtedly, the multifaceted differentiation- and individualization possibilities available with the materials will require of the teacher that he/she shows a consistently high degree of presence in the remedial training situation. He/she must comprehensively structure the training events, varying them in a targeted manner as well. What is required of him/her for that purpose, is professional competence and far-reaching socio-emotional aptitudes, both of which render the successful use of the materials possible at all in the first place (Darch and Kam'enui, 2004; Larkin and Ellis, 2004; Scott, 1999) – i.e. changes in the students' critical competencies which can be brought about with the materials will vitally depend upon the conceptual orientations and the teacher's courses of educational action practically possible. A remedial training merely limiting itself to a mechanical "execution" or "realization" of the materials presented will render the approach ineffective at best.

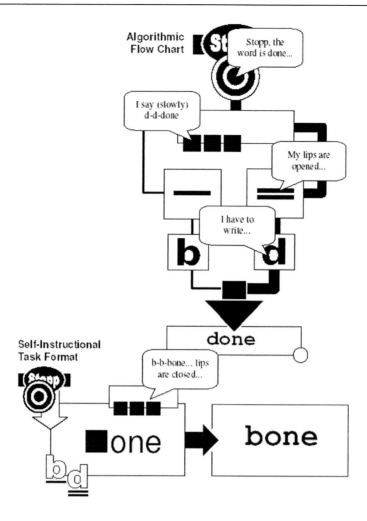

Figure 8. Algorithmic flow chart and task format concerning phonological skills (Faber, 2005b): An English worded example

EMPIRICAL FINDINGS

Treatment and Evaluation Setting

The systematic work with graphic algorithms and verbal self-instructions has been developed and tested in the extracurricular training of dyslexic students over many years. Within this approach, children and adolescents of any grade and educational level are instructed and looked after. These students are permanently unable to meet the reading and spelling demands in school despite additional spelling interventions, and they increasingly react to their persistent failures in a socio-emotionally noticeable way. In all cases examined, the intervention consisted of an individually compiled sequence of specific learning steps pertaining to the kind of errors in different orthographic domains, exclusively and intensely using visualized problem-solving algorithms and verbal self-instructions. Predominantly, this concerned the spelling skill areas of explosive consonant graphemes (gk/dt/bp), elongation/abbreviation (i/ie/ih, double consonants) und s-sounds (s/ss/ß). Within the single learning sequences, the command of orthographic rules required was first explored and worked out with the related problem-solving algorithms, and gradually consolidated with consistent referral to verbal self-instruction. According to the learning skill area, the partial skill components relevant to the analysis of speech sound length, derivation and/or elongation of words, syllable segmentation, and analysis of speech sound sharpness (acuity) were worked out and practiced. For the purpose of progressive habitualization of competencies worked out, and for the development of corresponding learning strategies, a learning program systematically tailored to the individual case with algorithmically formatted exercise materials, applicable in a self-instructive manner, was implemented (Faber, 2001b, 2002a,b, 2003a, 2004a,d). As of now, there are empirical findings from four training cohorts with dyslexic children and adolescents, with their remedial training spanning over a time period of 80 hours on an average – and with an analysis of their individual performance trends from beginning to end of the training (Studies 1 and 2). An additional study examines the development of orthographic competencies, comparing the results of trained and untrained students (Study 3).

Study 1

Evaluation Goals

For a first preliminary control of remedial training effects, the relevant spelling test data of three cohorts who had completed their remedial training were analyzed with regard to the performance improvements individually achieved (Faber, 2003b,c). The primary objective was to clarify whether the changes in orthographic competencies intraindividually achieved were distinctive enough overall so that they could not be attributed to random fluctuations or to errors in measurement, respectively – and thus could show at least a relative approximation of the students trained to the performance-related age norm. Another objective was to clarify whether the training methods and materials, applied in a relatively comparable way in all three cohorts, would lead to roughly similar results so that possible training effects would seem sufficiently reproducible and reliable from an intersubjective viewpoint as well. Accordingly, the following questions are supposed to be examined by this study:

- Is it possible to prove the evidence of significant performance gains on the part of the students in the cohorts trained?
- Has it been possible to observably approximate the performance of the students to those of their corresponding age norm?
- Do these effects turn out to be more or less equally strong in all training cohorts?

Subjects

The three cohorts examined consisted of overall 81 children and adolescents of different grade levels (Table 1) who displayed normal cognitive abilities (IQ $\geq$ 85) and showed extensive orthographic difficulties, in most cases already accumulated over a longer period of time. As variance analysis results showed, the composition of the cohorts did not differ significantly with regard to gender (F = 0.801, p = .495) nor grade level (F = 0.539, p = .656) nor the average duration of the training period (F = 1.220, p = .306). The analysis included only data of students whose performances in the spelling pre-test measure showed at least a standard deviation below their age-related norm. Moreover, it turned out that the students' orthographic difficulties could be associated, in the majority of cases, with inadequate (mostly impulsive, inactive and unfocused) learning styles, with strong motivational tendencies to avoid academic demands, as well as with frequently noticeable socio-emotional problems.

Basic Training Conditions

The intervention took place once a week for 60 minutes each in single individuals and/or in groups of two, spanning over a time period of 80 hours on an average. It was carried out by the author and another teacher who received regular consultation with regard to questions as to the didactic-methodical implementation of the approach. In addition, they introduced the fundamental procedures of spelling assessment, remedial training methods, as well as student-focused techniques of instructional work (Faber, 1991a).

Measurements and Statistical Analyses

Before and after the spelling training, the orthographic competencies of all students were assessed using standardized testing procedures. According to grade level, this happened with the WRT 2+ and the WRT 3+ (Birkel, 1994a,b), the DRT 4 and the DRT 5 (Grund, Haug and Naumann, 1994, 1995), the subtest A2 of the RST 6-7 (Rieder, 1984) or with the HSP 5-9 (May, 1998). For all data analyses, the students' test results were transformed into grade-related T score norms. The statistical examination of the performance effects of interest was carried out separately for each cohort using paired t-tests – with one-tailed questions and an alpha level of p < .05. For the supplementary evaluation of the relative performance gain, standardized effect sizes were calculated for each cohort as well (Cohen, 1988). The question of comparability of the three student groups among each other was checked for both measurement times using one-way analyses of variance (Peers, 1996).

Results

Prior to the spelling training, the orthographic performances of all three cohorts proved to be below average; after the training they reached an average competence level. Based on the relevant test norms, i.e. in the interindividual comparison to their peers, the children and adolescents trained were able to improve their performances by 1.5 standard deviations on an average. These performance changes can be clearly confirmed statistically for all cohorts as well (Table 1). Intraindividually, illustrated with the corresponding effect size, the relative performance gain in each cohort turned out to be even more succinct: as measured by the variance of the respective spelling test results prior to the training, the average rate of increase was clearly above 2 standard deviations. With all this, the cohorts did not differ significantly with regard to their performances, neither prior to the intervention nor afterwards. Corresponding one-way analyses of variance could not document significant differences in the pre-test (F = 1.247, p = .295), in the post-test (F = 0.618, p = .605) and in the pre-post-test figures (F = 1.104, p = .351) – i.e. all three cohorts had started the training with comparable pre-test performances and finished it with comparable achievement gains. However, the variances of the performance gains achieved in the cohorts also indicate that not all students benefited from the training to the same degree. On closer inspection of the relevant single-case data, some students can be found in every cohort whose performances showed an improvement of less than 10 T score points. These were mostly children and adolescents with relatively favorable test scores prior to the intervention which could suggest that a targeted training of these students might not have been necessary at all in the first place. Despite their orthographic competencies ranging close to the average, the students showed consistently weak results in the class dictation (with up to 20 word errors) prior to the intervention. Discrepancies of this kind with regard to competence and performance could essentially be traced back to massive test-anxious reactions and inadequate exercise practices. Meanwhile, the spelling training seems to have been successful in improving the motivational and strategic prerequisites for a more competent mastery of class dictations on the part of the students so that they all were able to significantly reduce their individual error ratios in the dictation after the training. In contrast, their final test results inevitably could reflect this development only to a limited degree.

Table 1. Spelling test performance in training cohorts 1, 2 and 3: comparison of pre- and post-test-data based on grade-referenced T scores norms (M = Mean, s = standard deviation, t = paired t-test , p = probability, d = effect size).

Training cohort 1 (1998/1999)								
8 females, 16 males: Grades 2 (n = 5), 3 (n = 3), 4 (n = 8), 5 (n = 6), 6 (n = 2)								
Training time: 81 hours in average								
Pre-test		Post-test		Difference				
M	s	M	s	M	s	t	p	d
32	4.5	47	6.0	+15	6.0	12.479	.0000	2.50

Training cohort 2 (1999/2000)								
5 females, 26 males: Grades 3 (n = 10), 4 (n = 7), 5 (n = 10), 6 (n = 4)								
Training time: 80 hours in average								
Pre-test		Post-test		Difference				
M	s	M	s	M	s	t	p	d
35	4.8	50	6.5	+15	6.4	13.269	.0000	2.34

Training cohort 3 (2000/2001)								
9 females, 17 males: Grades 3 (n = 7), 4 (n = 4), 5 (n = 12), 7 (n = 3)								
Training time: 82 hours in average								
Pre-test		Post-test		Difference				
M	s	M	s	M	s	t	p	d
34	6.6	51	4.2	+17	8.2	10.347	.0000	2.07

Discussion

The empirical analysis of three different cohorts of dyslexic children and adolescents whose training included systematic use of visualized problem-solving algorithms and verbal self-instructions over a longer period of time was able to prove consistent and significant gains in spelling test performance. Interindividually, the mostly below-average pre-test scores could be nominally improved up to an average level of competence, with a comparable development of all cohorts trained. Intraindividually, as proven by the corresponding effect sizes, the improvements in students' spelling test performance achieved turn out to be very significant from the practical viewpoint as well. The strikingly high effect sizes could have been the result, last but not least, of the relatively little variances observed in the pre-post-test differences. However, this circumstance clearly shows that the remedial training of the cohorts which were quite heterogeneous within themselves must have realized a sufficient degree of educational individualization and adaptation.

Study 2

Evaluation Goals

With another evaluation setting, the objective of the study was to find out whether the performance gains achieved in the cohorts trained up to that point could be replicated with other cohorts – at the same time however, they were also supposed to contribute to rendering the findings hitherto compiled more precise (Faber, 2004b): as such, the potential influence of statistical regression tendencies on the changes in the students' spelling test performances in the previous study has not been taken into consideration yet. However, as the dyslexic student cohorts trained in particular show, by definition, extremely low pre-test scores, representing a negatively selected sample, it cannot be ruled out that corresponding regression effects have had an influence on the pre-post-test comparisons conducted, possibly having contributed, to a certain degree, to a relative overestimation of the performance changes registered. Regression effects of that kind become statistically controllable when the differences in the test scores between two measurement times are known before an independent intervention variable on the feature of interest has taken place. In case of substantial regression tendencies, the first measurement would have to be correlated negatively with the difference between first and subsequent measurements (Rogosa and Willett, 1985). For this reason, the research design was supplemented with an additional measurement time with spelling test data collected about four months prior to the beginning of the training. The comparison of both test scores – which of course cannot reflect effects resulting from the intervention yet – should provide sufficiently confirmed clues and leads for measuring the degree of changes in the students' performances depending on regression effects. In addition, the evaluation of training effects after completion of the intervention encounters tight limitations with regard to sounding the performance development of the individually trained students by comparing trained and untrained learning skill areas – insofar as the training concept to be evaluated per se provides for the systematic handling of all critical spelling aspects. Therefore, respective error-specific evaluation efforts can only ask for differences between systematically trained spelling skill areas and those incidentally considered. Thus, the research design of this study analyzed the performance development predominantly in the systematically trained spelling skill areas explosive consonant graphemes (gk/dt/bp), i-graphemes (i/ie/ih) as well as doubling of consonants and s-graphemes (s/ss/ß) which all students had worked on, in their entirety, in separate training sequences, systematically applying the concept-specific methods and materials. As additional control criteria, the research design also took the performances in spelling skill areas capitalization and phonologically based spelling into consideration which the students had not worked on in separate training units – the mastery of which the students nevertheless had to engage in implicitly while dealing with their respective training contents, and which had to be purposefully supported in the training if necessary. In this way, the study was supposed to yield significant clues and leads as to whether the advancements in the students' performances remained mostly limited to the systematically trained spelling skill areas, or if they could be generally verified across all spelling skill areas. However, the empirical findings with regard to the evaluation of orthographic rule training do not imply general transfer effects (Mannhaupt, 2003; Scheerer-Neumann, 1993). Another aspect of the transfer of training effects concerns the changes achieved which are relatively independent from the responsible teachers. Undoubtedly, the suitability of a training concept depends to a large degree on the aspect that different users arrive at relatively comparable results under similar circumstances, provided that the concept-specific training instructions are being adhered to in a reliable way. Therefore, the research design also included an examination of the students' performances with regard to their respective teacher. In this sense, the performance data of the student cohort studied were supposed to be analyzed in detail, considering the following questions:

- Do the students' spelling test scores increase, already prior to the beginning of the training, to such a degree – depending upon regression effects – that it would suggest the exclusive use of the data collected at the time of the second measurement for a methodically sufficient study of performance changes resulting from the intervention?
- Is it possible to demonstrate statistically and practically significant improvements in the individual students' spelling test performances near the end of the training in a pre-post-test comparison, both on a broad basis of total test scores as well as
- specifically in the three systematically trained spelling skill areas?
- By comparison, do possible advancements in the two spelling skill areas incidentally considered turn out to be relatively little or completely insignificant?
- Do the students' performances achieved near the end of the training differ significantly, subject to the teacher responsible in each respective case?

Subjects

The cohort examined in this study was comprised of 19 boys of different grade levels who displayed normal cognitive abilities but had extensive orthographic difficulties which, in most cases, had already been accumulated over a longer period of time. A third of them (33%) had already participated in school-based remediation activities for more than a year, almost half of them (48%) for nearly a year. As variance analysis results could show, there were no differences in their performance with regard to the duration of their previous training ($F = 0.711$, $p = .504$). Detailed spelling error analyses revealed clear evidence, that the students' orthographic difficulties could be traced back to a lack of rule-dependent competencies and strategies in most cases – violations of the phonologically based spelling of words were relatively rare overall (Table 3). In the majority of cases, the performance problems were associated with inadequate (mostly impulsive, inactive and unfocused) learning styles, motivational orientations characterized by test anxiety and avoidant behaviors, as well as socio-emotional conspicuities in a large number of cases. According to reports from parents, severe conflicts with regard to homework and additional domestic exercise attempts were arising frequently. The lack of autonomy, the inability to stay focused on the task, as well as partially aggressive avoidance reactions on the part of the children and adolescents were considered particularly critical.

Basic Training Conditions

In all cases studied, the spelling training consisted of an individually compiled sequence of area-specific training steps addressing different orthographic problems with extensive use of visualized problem-solving algorithms and verbal self-instructions – in the majority of cases, this concerned the spelling skill areas explosive consonant graphemes (gk/dt/bp), i-graphemes (i/ie/ih), as well as doubling of consonants and s-graphemes (s/ss/ß). In contrast, the incidentally considered spelling skill area capitalization was only picked out as a central theme in cases of individual uncertainties or errors; the students were then supposed to show the critical front part of the word with the aid of a corresponding signal card and by thinking aloud (Faber, 2004c). Similarly, the incidentally considered skill area of phonologically based spelling was picked out as a central theme as required, by also focusing the students' attention on the critical work part with signal cards, and getting them to think aloud about their spelling activities. Often this concerned problems around the subjects of differentiating sounds and, in particular, structuring or segmenting words – the mastery of which is, with elaborate syllablization exercises, already a central component part of the spelling strategies imparted in the training units dealing with explosive sounds and doubling of consonants. The intervention took place once a week for 60 minutes each with single individuals and/or groups of two. It was carried out by the author and another teacher who received regular consultation with regard to questions as to the diagnostic and methodical implementation of the approach.

Measurements and Statistical Analyses

The students' orthographic achievement were first recorded in pre-test 1 four months prior, on an average, to the beginning of the intervention (AM = 4.3, s = 0.9), and again in pre-test 2 directly at the beginning of the intervention, as well as in subsequent follow-up tests after 40 hours into the training, and in the post-test near the end of the training, each time with standardized testing procedures. According to grade level, this took place with the WRT 2+ and the WRT 3+ (Birkel, 1994a,b), the DRT 4 and the DRT 5 (Grund, Haug and Naumann, 1994, 1995), the subtest A2 of the RST 6-7 (Rieder, 1984) or with the HSP 5-9 (May, 1998). In pre-test 2, it was possible to use parallel forms of the instruments employed in pre-test 1. Due to the training spanning over quite a long time period, as follow-up and post-test measures instruments with norms for the next higher grade level were administered in each case. Evaluation of test results was carried out quantitatively on the basis of grade-related T score norms, as well as qualitatively with the proviso of descriptive error categories. For this purpose, error percentage values were generated, qualifying the individual appearance of orthographic rule violations with regard to the number of error-specific critical word parts in the respective spelling test. At the beginning of the treatment, the individual error rates in the various skill areas analyzed proved to be correlated only moderately (with r ranging from .01 to .45), so that it seemed sensible to prepare separate analyses for the systematically trained spelling skill areas explosive graphemes, i-graphemes and doubling of consonants/s-graphemes. Statistical examination of the performance effects of interest was carried out using paired t-tests with an (one-tailed) alpha error probability of $p < .05$. For the purpose of a supplementary assessment of the relative performance gains, standardized effect sizes were calculated as well (Cohen, 1988). The clarification of possible teacher-dependent effects on the students' performances was carried out for each measurement time using one-way analyses of variance with a two-tailed alpha error probability of p < .05 (Peers, 1996).

Results

The comparison to the spelling performances tested four months prior to the beginning of the treatment substantiates an average growth of 2.6 T score points (from M_1 = 33.6 to M_2 = 36.2). At the same time, the results of pre-test 1 turned out to be correlated to the difference between pre-test 1 and 2 with r = -.62 (p = .005), i.e. students with extremely low initial test scores in particular show increased performances due to statistical regression tendencies. This effect can not influence the students' interindividual achievement differences, insofar as both test scores proved to be highly correlated (r = .94, p = .000) – however, it corrected the initial level of orthographic achievement for the entire cohort in a significant way upwards (t = -5.843, p = .000). The analysis of treatment effects must make allowances for this circumstance in that the spelling test scores from pre-test 2, statistically controlled for regression effects, are to be used exclusively as the methodically more solid criterion for the evaluation of the students' performances prior to the beginning of the training. Under these circumstances, the spelling test performances, prior to the training, of the cohort examined turned out to be below average and improved temporarily by 11 T score points on an average at the time of the follow-up measurement, and by 12 T score points at the time of post-test measurement. The extent of changes intraindividually achieved hereby can be statistically confirmed for the students, and due to the respective effect sizes it can be considered very important in practical terms as well. Intraindividually, therefore in alignment with the respective test norms, the average growth rate near the end of the treatment amounts to more than one standard deviation (Table 2). There were no substantial correlations between the extent of performance gains, i.e. the difference between the results in pre-test 2 and in the post-test, and the grade level (r = -.18, p > .05). Obviously, the students' age and the extend of their individual school experiences already did not play a crucial role with regard to their spelling improvements. The fact that the students' performance gains from pre-test 2 to post-test turned out to be considerably stronger than those from pre-test 1 to pre-test 2, reveals strong evidence for the remedial efficacy of the spelling training.

At the same time, the trend of all performance data points up a strikingly distinctive pattern (Figure 9): the orthographic performances, extremely weak at first, tend to increase significantly by the time halfway into the training. However, until the end of the treatment, this growth does not continue at the same rate; it rather seems that the performance level achieved remains more or less the same. Obviously, the development of competencies seems to stagnate throughout the second half of the treatment. However, as the grade-related T score norms near the end of the intervention reflect the increased demands of the next higher grade level in each case, the students' competencies between the third and fourth measuring time might have increased in actual fact.

Table 2. Spelling test performance in training cohort 4: comparison of pre-test, follow-up, and post-test data based on grade-referenced T scores norms (M = Mean, s = standard deviation, t = paired t-test , p = probability, d = effect size)

Training cohort 4 (2002/2003)
19 males: Grades 2 (n = 1), 3 (n = 2), 4 (n = 10), 5 (n = 1), 6 (n = 3), 7 (n = 2)
Total training time: 90 hours in average

Pre-test		Follow-up		Difference				
M	s	M	s	M	s	t	p	d
36.2	3.3	47.5	5.0	+11.3	4.6	10.746	.0000	2.46

Follow-up		Post-test		Difference				
M	s	M	S	M	s	t	p	d
47.5	5.0	48.8	5.4	+1.3	4.1	1.405	.0089	0.32

Pre-test		Post-test		Difference				
M	s	M	s	M	s	t	p	d
36.2	3.3	48.8	5.4	+12.6	5.7	9.621	.0000	2.21

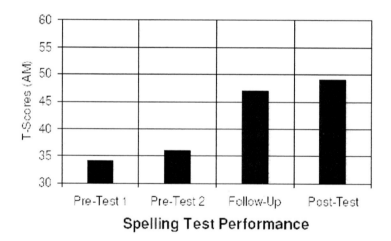

Spelling Test Performance

Figure 9. Development of spelling competencies in training cohort 4: Norm-referenced spelling test scores 4 months prior to the training (pre-test 1), at the beginning of the training (pre-test 2), after 40 hours of training time (follow-up), and at the end of the training after 80 hours (post-test)

The results in the systematically trained spelling skill areas present themselves in similar ways (Table 3). In both areas, explosive und i-graphemes, as well as in the area doubling of consonants/s-graphemes, the average error rates have decreased to an extent which, due to its consistently high statistical significance, has to be regarded as very important in practical terms. The area-specific differences between the students at the beginning of the treatment could evidently be reduced. However, remarkable gains in performance can also be found in the incidentally considered spelling skill areas. As could be expected, they turn out to be not quite as significant, by comparison, but still momentous in statistical and practical terms.

Overall, the average error rate in the areas capitalization and phonologically based spelling has reduced significantly. At the same time, the performance gains in phonologically based spelling do not seem to have come about independent from changes in the systematically trained spelling skill area explosive consonant graphemes. Because, near the end of the intervention the two error percentage rates correlate to r = .62 (p = .006) more strongly than prior to the beginning of the treatment when the respective relationship amounted to r = -.01 (p =. 984) – i.e. those students in particular who were able to significantly increase their competencies in the area of explosive consonant graphemes also showed improved performances in the area of phonologically based spelling.

Table 3. Error rates in various spelling skill areas: comparison of pre- and post-test data in training cohort 4 (M = Mean, s = standard deviation, t = paired t-test, p = probability, d = effect size)

Error rates in spelling skill area gk+ (systematically trained)								
Pre-test		Post-test		Difference				
M	s	M	s	M	s	t	p	d
19.0	14.1	4.9	4.0	-14.1	13.6	4.518	.0000	1.04
Error rates in spelling skill area ieih (systematically trained)								
Pre-test		Post-test		Difference				
M	s	M	s	M	s	t	p	d
25.8	15.0	5.5	6.1	-20.3	13.7	6.462	.0000	1.48
Error rates in spelling skill area IIss (systematically trained)								
Pre-test		Post-test		Difference				
M	s	M	s	M	s	t	p	d
38.8	21.1	12.3	8.9	-26.5	20.0	5.769	.0000	1.33
Error rates in spelling skill area grokl (incidentally trained)								
Pre-test		Post-test		Difference				
M	s	M	s	M	s	t	p	d
14.6	11.0	4.4	3.9	-10.2	10.4	4.284	.0000	0.98
Error rates in spelling skill area lautg (incidentally trained)								
Pre-test		Post-test		Difference				
M	s	M	s	M	s	t	p	d
7.7	5.9	3.4	2.6	-4.3	4.9	3.751	.0010	0.88

Spelling skill areas: gk+ = explosive consonant graphemes (gk, dt, bp), ieih = i-graphemes, IIss = double consonants and s-graphemes, grokl = capitalization rules, lautg = phonologically based spelling (phoneme-grapheme correspondences)

In addition, a certain pattern of area-related progression becomes apparent across all three measurement times (Figure 10). In the first half of the intervention, the error rates, both in the systematically trained and the incidentally considered spelling skill areas, tend to be reduced significantly. This trend then tends to level out notedly near the end of the treatment – the extent of relative performance gains is less prominent.

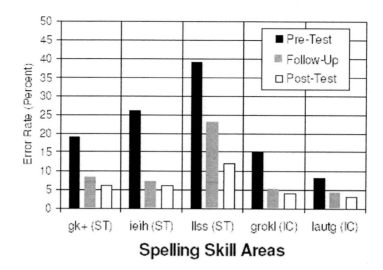

Spelling Skill Areas

Figure 10. Error rates in various spelling skill areas: Pre-test, follow-up, and post-test data in training cohort 4 (gk+ = explosive consonant graphemes, ieih = i-graphemes, IIss = doubling of consonants and s-graphemes, grokl = capitalization, lautg = phonologically based spelling, ST = systematically trained, IC = indicentally considered)

With all this, it is not possible to eventually prove the evidence of significant differences, in terms of variance analysis results, in the students' performances near the end of the treatment which could be traced back in any way to the teaching persons (Table 4). Under the basic reserve that different teachers do not necessarily arrive at completely identical results even when the working conditions are the same, no significant teacher effects can be identified at any measurement time. The dyslexic students and adolescents were assigned to both teachers exclusively according to the chronological sequence of their registration for the treatment; they start the training with largely comparable performance characteristics, and they complete it with largely similar performance characteristics. The differences existing in the students' post-test results still turned out to be insignificant in statistical terms.

Table 4. Teacher-dependent differences in spelling test performance of training cohort 4: comparisons of pre-test, follow-up, and post-test data based on grade-referenced T score norms (M = Mean, s = standard deviation, df = degrees of freedom, F = F ratio of variance analysis, d = effect size)

	Teacher A		Teacher B				
	n = 8 students		n = 11 students				
	M	s	M	s	df	F	p
Pre-test	35.4	3.7	36.8	2.9	1,17	0.903	.355
Follow-up	45.1	3.5	49.1	5.4	1,17	3.388	.083
Post-test	46.1	4.4	50.7	5.4	1,17	3.905	.065

Discussion

The evaluation of training a cohort consisting of male dyslexic students over a time period of nearly two years by systematically using algorithmic problem-solving plans and verbal self-instructions, shows consistently significant improvements in the students' orthographic competencies. Both on the basis of pertinent test norms, and in the error percentage values of the systematically trained spelling skill areas, a significantly reduced extent of orthographic rule violations can be identified – inter- and intraindividually. At the same time, a consistent pattern of progression becomes apparent in the training, insofar as the students are at first able to considerably increase their performances – very poor in the beginning – and then maintaining the improvement at a stable level. In the incidentally considered spelling skill areas students have made progress as well – not as significant, by comparison, but still to a considerable extent. To what extent this result is to be understood as a long-term consequence of a strategic transfer when it comes to the area of capitalization – which was merely discussed, if necessary, by thinking-aloud application of a corresponding signal card – can only be assumed for the time being. Possibly, the rule-specific work with algorithmic problem-solving patterns has led to a more conscious perception and a more consistent analysis of speech or language structural work characteristics on the part of the students in general, so that the habitualization of respective cognitive concepts of problem-solving has been supported by regular use of the signal card, having facilitated the generalization of strategically beneficial behavioral patterns. In similar ways, although less clearly traceable as to content and method, the performance gains in phonologically spelling skills can be explained: here in particular, the consistent training of rule-specific partial competencies in the spelling skill area explosive consonant graphemes, namely the syllablizing segmentation of elongated word forms, seems to have been crucial in reducing phonologically based misspellings. Comparable transfer effects could already be proved elsewhere (Tacke, Wörner and Brezing, 1993) – however, predominantly with the proviso that syllablizing speech exercises can have a beneficial effect on phonological and orthographical, therefore rule-specific orthographic competencies as well. With the results at hand, the question about such transfer effects can of course be reversed and expanded, insofar as the use of rule-specific syllablization exercises can also result in general improvements in the students' phonological performances. In methodical terms, the consideration of both effect directions could provide additional starting points for a far-reaching integration of phonologically and rule-specific treatment components geared to the learning requirements of each individual case (Blachman, Schatschneider, Fletcher, Francis, Clonan, Shaywitz and Shaywitz, 2004; 2000; Lovett, Lacerenza, Borden, Frijters, Steinbach and De Palma, 2000; Weber, Marx and Schneider, 2002). The results of the study at hand – which took into concentration the students' performance changes depending on regression effects prior to the beginning of the training for the first time – certainly qualify the findings from previous effect analyses in retrospection, insofar as the pre-post-test differences in the spelling norm scores reported there could be foreseen as slightly overestimated. The efficiency of the training approach, proven across the boards, does not seem to be called into question at all thereby. Because the results of this evaluation study, on the basis of performance figures statistically controlled for regression effects, confirm in any case the results and findings for the evaluation of rule-oriented and/or strategy-oriented interventions. Of course, it is imperative to replicate and specify these results and findings as well. In doing so, future evaluation settings should replace in particular the test-dependent percentage values, calculated so far, for the purpose of compiling the area-specific error ratios, with more suitable criteria in terms of content and psychometry (Klicpera and Gasteiger-Klicpera, 1995). For this purpose, a standardized word list in two parallel forms exists in the meantime which can serve to register and analyze, with regard to spelling area and/or strategy, the students' orthographic competencies in the selected skill areas such as explosive consonant graphemes, i-graphemes, doubling of consonants, and s-graphemes (Faber, 2004d). And finally, this study could provide the first evidences that the students' performance advancements achieved were relatively independent from the person of the teacher. Therefore, it seems possible for different users, at least on the proviso that the training of the dyslexic students and the counseling of the remedial teachers are consistently being accompanied in practice (Faber, 2003a), to arrive at roughly comparable treatment results in similar work contexts if the concept-specific training instructions are being adhered to.

Study 3

Evaluation Goals

With the third evaluation setting, the objective was to analyze the temporary effects on spelling performance in a fifth training cohort, and to compare it with the performance changes in a corresponding control group of students not (yet) trained. On the basis of the results hitherto existing, it was expected that the students of the conceptually trained experimental group would show significantly better post-test results, given roughly similar pre-test performances, than the students of the untrained control group – both on the basis of general test norm scores and with respect to trained and untrained spelling skill areas selected. For that purpose, the relative error rates in three systematically trained skill areas which all students in the experimental group worked on in separate training units, systematically applying the concept-specific methods and materials in their entirety, are used as area-specific performance criteria. Moreover, the performances in two learning fields not addressed with separate training units – which nevertheless had to be mastered by the students though, in dealing with their respective training contents, and which had to be supported in a targeted way if necessary – were used as additional control criteria. And finally, the performances in two completely untrained skill areas were taken into consideration. A superiority of the experimental group by comparison, in these untrained fields in particular, could indicate potential strategic transfer effects as a result of the intervention (Klauer, 2000). However, the empirical findings with regard to the effectiveness of orthographic rule training could not really prove general transfer effects of this kind up to now (Mannhaupt, 2003; Scheerer-Neumann, 1993). Accordingly, the general and error-specific orthographic competencies of both student groups were examined, taking the following questions into consideration:

- Is it possible to establish and demonstrate in the post-test overall significantly better orthographic performances in the experimental group, compared to the students in the control group?
- Is it possible to establish and demonstrate in the post-test significantly lower error rates in three systematically trained spelling skill areas in the experimental group, compared to the students in the control group?
- Is it possible to establish and demonstrate in the post-test significantly lower error rates in two incidentally considered spelling skill areas in the experimental group, compared to the students in the control group?

- Is it possible to establish and demonstrate in the post-test significantly lower error rates in two untrained spelling skill areas in the experimental group, compared to the students in the control group?

Subjects

The students selected for both the experimental and the control group displayed normal cognitive abilities (average IQ: 102) as well as extensive and, in most cases, rule-specific orthographic difficulties accumulated over a longer time period which could not be significantly reduced despite regular school training – so a pertinent extracurricular treatment seemed urgently advisable. In most cases, their orthographic difficulties could be traced back to a lack of plain orthographic knowledge and solution strategies. The performance problems turned out to be associated, to a large extent, with inadequate (mostly impulsive, inactive, and inattentive) learning styles, with unfavourable motivational orientations, as well as with distinctive socio-emotional characteristics in many cases. The experimental group was comprised of 8 boys and 10 girls who had already participated in the intervention for 34 hours. The untrained control group consisted of 11 boys and 7 girls with an average waiting period of 8 months (SD = 1.39). Both student groups did not differ significantly from each other, neither with regard to gender (t = 0.987, df = 33.9, p = .331) nor with regard to grade level (t = 0.908, df = 33.9, p = .370). With respect to the initial performances in the orthographic test however, a slight advantage for the students in the experimental group became apparent, the extent of which proved to be significant (t = 2.457, df = 34, p = .019). Moreover, with the students in the control group it was not possible to establish a significant correlation with regard to their orthographic performance and their participation in school-based training: the duration of their regular school training hitherto completed turned out to be correlated with their pre-test performances by r = -.16 (p = .586) and with their post-test performances by r = -.15 (p = .614). It was not possible either to establish a significant correlation between pre-test and post-test performances with the parents' evaluation of regular school training effects (Faber, 2003d). Here, the corresponding correlations amounted to r = .05 and r = -.03 (p > .05). In this respect, possible influences of the regular spelling school training on the performance changes examined could be ruled out to a large extent.

Measurements and Statistical Analyses

The spelling performances of the students in the experimental group were recorded at measurement time 1 (pre-test) directly at the beginning of the treatment, as well as that measurement time 2 after 34 hours into the training (post-test), with standardized testing procedures. For the students in the control group, the performance assessment was carried out analogously at measurement time 1 (pre-test) about eight months prior to the beginning of the treatment, and at measurement time 2 (post-test) directly at its beginning. According to grade level, this happened for all students with the WRT 3+ (Birkel, 1994b), the DRT 4, and the DRT 5 (Grund, Haug and Naumann, 1994, 1995), the subtest A2 of the RST 6-7 (Rieder, 1984), or with the HSP 5-9 (May, 1998). At measurement time 2, the procedure for the next higher grade was used in each case. Evaluation of the test results was carried out quantitatively on the basis of grade-related T score norms. In addition, at measurement time 2 a especially developed word list was used to establish the students' error-specific competencies in the spelling skill areas explosive consonant graphemes (25 word parts with gk/dt/bp), i-graphemes (16 word parts with i/ie/ih), doubling of consonants (26 word parts including ck and tz), as well as s-graphemes (15 word parts with s/ss/ß) on the basis of 60 word dictations in each case (Faber, 2004d). The individual frequency of error-specific orthographic rule violations is relativized by the number of critical word parts appearing in the list for each learning field, and it is converted into corresponding error percentage scores. Overall, this procedure promises, as to content and psychometry, more adequate results with regard to the students' individual error ratio, as these are not any longer directly depending upon the item pool of a certain spelling test. For all students in the experimental and control groups (N = 36), the internal consistency of the word list amounted to α = .93 (Cronbach's Alpha). The sum total of list words correctly written correlated with the T score norms of the spelling test procedures by r = .56 (p = .005) and turned out to be significantly influenced by the grade level (r = .55, p = .007) but not by gender (r = .01, p > .05). Due to the previous course of the training, the corresponding error percentage scores in the areas explosive consonant graphemes, i-graphemes and doubling of consonants were used, for the study at hand, as error-specific performance criteria for the systematically trained skill areas – and the error percentage scores in capitalization and phonologically based spelling were used as error-specific performance criteria in the incidentally considered skill areas. The error percentage scores in the untrained skill areas s-graphemes and eä/fv-graphemes served as additional control criteria. The calculation of the eä/fv errors still had to be dependent upon the corresponding item pools of the test procedures used. As children and adolescents with localized orthographic difficulties in particular tend to several misspellings in one single word often, the ordinary test sum scores can, foreseeably, only roughly reflect the extent of their individual difficulties. Therefore, their individual error frequency was recorded as an additional performance criterion, relativizing the sum total of individual errors in the spelling test with the total item sum of the corresponding procedure (Valtin, Badel, Löffler, Meyer-Schepers and Voss, 2003). With the test norm scores, the error frequency of all students at measurement time 1 correlated to r = -.81 (p = .000), as was expected. The spelling performances of all students were recorded at two different measurement times. The time span in between them amounted to 34 weeks in the experimental group and 32 weeks in the control group. To clarify possible performance differences due to treatment, the spelling test performances of the students in both groups were first of all compared with the paired t-test at measurement time 2 – using one-tailed questions with a predefined alpha error probability of p < .05. The extent of these differences were quantified via corresponding effect sizes, with the post-test differences of both groups relativized with their common (pooled) variances in performance, and additionally adjusted with respect to possible pre-test effects (Peers, 1996; Masendorf, 1997). In similar ways, the study of error-specific performance differences between students in both groups at measurement time 2 was conducted, as well the analysis of the performance level in the systematically trained, the incidentally considered, and the untrained spelling skill areas. In addition, the differences between measurement times 2 and 1 that showed up in each group were subjected to a statistical inspection using paired t-tests. For the purpose of an additional evaluation of relative performance gains, standardized effect sizes were calculated (Cohen, 1988).

Basic Training Conditions

For the students in the experimental group, the training up to measurement time 2 (post-test) consisted of an individually compiled sequence of error-specific learning sequences addressing different orthographic problems, making extensive use of visualized problem-solving algorithms and verbal self-instructions – in particular in the spelling skill areas explosive consonant graphemes, i-graphemes and doubling of consonants. In the single learning unit of these systematically trained skill areas, the necessary knowledge of orthographic rules was systematically explored and developed, at first with the respective problem-solving algorithms, and then gradually consolidated with the consistent use of verbal self-instructions. According to each skill area, the solution-relevant partial competencies with regard to analysis of sound length, flection/elongation of words, and syllable segmentization, were worked out and practiced. For the purpose of a progressive habitualization of these competencies, an individually tailored learning program with algorithmically formatted practice materials, applicable in a self-instructive way, was implemented in each case. In contrast, the incidentally considered spelling skill area capitalization was only discussed in the case of individual uncertainties or errors, and the students were then supposed to indicate the critical beginning of the word with a corresponding single card by thinking aloud. Similarly, the incidentally considered spelling skill area phonologically based spelling was discussed in case of need, by also directing the students' attention to the critical word part and prompting them to examine their spelling activities by thinking aloud (Faber, 2004c). Often this addressed problems pertaining to word segmentation – the mastery of which is already a central component part of the spelling strategies conveyed in the systematically trained skill areas explosive consonant graphemes and doubling of consonants by applying meticulous syllablization exercises. Critical words from the two untrained spelling skill areas s-graphemes and eä/fv-graphemes were not addressed directly but rather collected in a corresponding learning card index file and written in regular intervals. The training was carried out once a week for 60 minutes each in single sessions. It was conducted by the author exclusively.

Results

The spelling test performances of the students in the control group had improved at measurement time 2 by 2.6 (SD = 2.3) from 31.3 to 33.9 T score points (t = -4.755, df = 17, p = .000) on an average. This change already proved to be statistically significant and, with a relative effect size of d = 1.11 practically momentous as well; *interindividually* however, it still turns out to be inadequate. The surprisingly high effect size can be primarily explained, though, with the small variance in the pre-post-test differences of the test scores, which results in the fact that even relatively small performance gains are inevitably overestimated – and that the effect size calculated rather reflects the homogeneity of the control group than a change in the students' achievement. This circumstance also becomes obvious by the fact that the initial performances of the students in the control group correlated to their pre-post-test differences only by r = -.03 (p = .452) overall. Therefore, the performance changes in the control group cannot be attributed, statistically and reliably, to a possible regression effect either. In contrast, the performances of the students in the experimental group at measurement time 2 temporarily improved, on an average, by 11.3 (SD = 4.4) from 34.6 to 45.8 T score points. The extent of changes intraindividually achieved therewith can be statistically confirmed (t = -10.801, df = 17, p = .000), and with a relative effect size of d = 2.55 it can also be considered very important in practical terms. At the same time, this change also seems significant in an intraindividual frame of reference. As the pre-post-test differences in the experimental group clearly show a wider variance than in the control group, the effect size calculated seems to be overestimated, foreseeably, to a lesser extent. Accordingly, the spelling performances of the students in the experimental group at measurement time 2 appear far superior (Figure 11): the median performance differences between both groups amounted to 11.9 T score points and proves to be highly significant (t = 8.289, df = 34, p = .000). At measurement time 2, the relative performance gain of the students in the experimental group amounts to more than two standard deviations of the overall achievement variance. The corresponding effect size amounts to d = 2.76 (Peers, 1996). If this value is adjusted, taking the influence of possible pre-test effects into consideration, then the relative effect size reduces itself to d_{corr} = 1.90 (Masendorf, 1997) – which does not substantially reduce the practical significance of the performance improvement, though. With all this, the extent of the previous performance gains in the experimental group, i.e. the difference between measurement time 1 and 2, turns out not to be significantly influenced by the grade level (Kruskal-Wallis test: chi square = 4.119, df = 4, p = .390). According to that, age and number of years already in school did not play any noteworthy role with respect to the performance changes achieved. Likewise, it is not possible to establish gender-specific differences (paired t-test: t = -1.722, df = 16, p = .104).

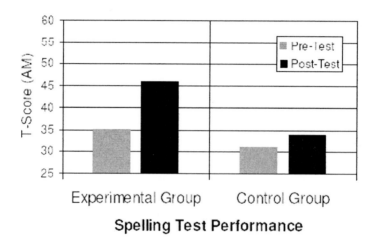

Figure 11. Comparison of pre- and post-test spelling test performances in the experimental and control group

With respect to the single spelling skill areas, this profound difference in performance between the students in the experimental group and those in the control group is stated more precisely (Table 5): at measurement time 2, the students in the experimental group show significantly lower error rates in the three systematically trained skill areas explosive consonant graphemes, i-graphemes, and doubling of consonants than the students in the control group. The same goes for the incidentally considered skill areas capitalization and phonologically based spelling. But their error rate is also significantly lower in the untrained skill areas s-graphemes and eä/fv-graphemes. In the majority of cases, the error-specific performances in the experimental group, compared with the control group, vary significantly less – i.e. it was obviously possible to reduce the respective interindividual differences among the trained students. The superiority of the students in the experimental group can be sufficiently confirmed in statistical terms and is to be considered as very significant in practical terms – insofar as its extent is lying consistently above a standard deviation of the common characteristics variances. In addition, the students in the experimental group were able to significantly reduce and even halve their individual error frequency which amounted to an average value of 96% prior to the treatment.

Table 5. Overall and area-specific error rates: comparison of post-test data between experimental and control group students (M = Mean, s = standard deviation, t = independent t-test, df = degrees of freedom, p = probability, d = effect size)

	Spelling skill area gk+ (systematically trained)					
	AM	s	t	df	p	d
Experimental group	9.3	7.1	-4.942	21.0	.0000	1.69
Control group	31.8	17.4				
	Spelling skill area ieih (systematically trained)					
	AM	S	t	df	p	d
Experimental group	10.3	9.5	-3.445	23.1	.0010	1.18
Control group	28.2	19.3				
	Spelling skill area ll+ (systematically trained)					
	AM	s	t	df	p	d
Experimental group	19.7	8.7	-3.655	22.6	.0005	1.25
Control group	37.5	18.2				
	Spelling skill area grokl (incidentally trained)					
	AM	s	t	df	p	d
Experimental group	5.6	3.1	-3.904	19.1	.0005	1.30
Control group	17.3	12.4				
	Spelling skill area lautg (incidentally trained)					
	AM	s	t	df	p	d
Experimental group	3.4	3.2	-3.599	17.6	.0010	1.20
Control group	24.2	24.3				
	Spelling skill area ssß (untrained)					
	AM	s	t	df	p	d
Experimental group	28.9	11.6	-2.838	20.1	.0050	1.03
Control group	48.0	23.6				
	Spelling skill area eäfv (untrained)					
	AM	s	t	df	p	d
Experimental group	23.1	19.1	-5.394	28.3	.0000	1.93
Control group	57.2	16.0				
	Overall error rate					
	AM	s	t	df	p	d
Experimental group	41.9	15.0	-6.161	20.1	.0000	2.04
Control group	115.9	52.6				

Spelling skill areas: gk+ = explosive consonant graphemes (gk, dt, bp), ieih = i-graphemes, ll+ = double consonants, ssß = s-graphemes, grokl = capitalization rules, lautg = phonologically based spelling (phoneme-grapheme correspondences), eäfv = eä- and fv-graphemes

Overall, at measurement time 2 (post-test) the performances in the experimental group across all spelling skill areas examined proved to be significantly better (Figure 12), compared to measurement time 1 (pre-test): the students were able to significantly reduce their individual error rates in the systematically trained spelling skill areas ($t = 7.003$, $p = 000$, $d = 1.81$) as well as in the incidentally considered skill areas ($t = 3.587$, $p = .003$, $d = 0.93$) and in the untrained skill areas ($t = 3.571$, $p = .006$, $d = 1.13$).

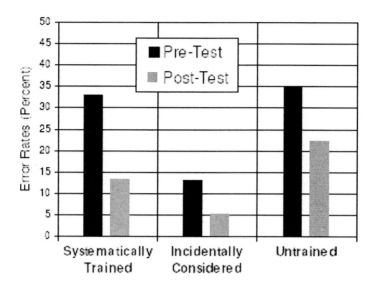

Figure 12. Performance gains in the experimental group's students: Comparison of error-rates in systematically trained, incidentally considered, and untrained spelling skill areas (Faber, 2005d)

Discussion

The study at hand can prove a significant superiority of the students in the experimental group who were conceptually trained, i.e. by systematically applying algorithmic and self-instructive task formats, with regard to their orthographic performances at measurement time 2, over the untrained students in the control group. After almost 8 months of training/waiting, the performance gains achieved by the students in the experimental group turns out to be statistically significant and practically relevant, both at the level of test norm scores and at the level of individual error frequencies. The analysis of the differences in performance between both groups at measurement time 1 does not make less of the fact either that the effect observed remains substantial. At the same time, the advances made in the experimental group could be brought about largely independent from the students' gender and grade level. The age-related heterogeneity of both student groups does reflect the actual circumstances of the respective practical intervention and thus lends support to the external validity of the evaluation setting – however, it should have had a foreseeably limiting effect its internal validity. Viewed in this way, future complementary training studies should be conducted on a broader sample basis with, among others, a better control of the student samples participating with regard to how they come into being and how they are composed. Under this reserve, the results of the study at hand do not only prove a general performance advance of the experimental group, but with respect to all spelling skill areas analyzed, they illustrate their consistent superiority over the control group: as could be expected, the orthographic competencies of the conceptually trained students in both the systematically trained and the incidentally considered skill areas proved to be significantly better. But the significant performance improvements of the experimental group also show up in the two untrained skill areas. While the changes achieved in the systematically trained skill areas can be foreseeably considered as direct effects of the respective area-specific intervention, the improvements in the other skill areas can be most likely explained with relevant transfer effects – in two ways: as such, it can be assumed that the advances in the incidentally considered skill area phonologically based spelling might have come about by the transfer of syllablizing strategies which were systematically developed and consolidated in connection with the explosive consonant graphemes and the doubling of consonants. The fact that the students' performances in the skill areas explosive consonant sounds and phonologically based spelling correlated significantly higher at measurement time 2 than at measurement time 1 might be at least an indicator for such an effect (Faber, 2005d). Accordingly, a strategically successful transfer of basic competencies, area-specifically practiced, to different orthographic cases of application could be assumed. Whether the improvements in the likewise incidentally considered skill area field capitalization can be traced back predominantly to the consistent use of the corresponding signal card and/or to strategic transfer effects, has to be left unanswered for the time being. It is possible that the algorithmic and self-instructive approach contributed to a more conscious observance of structural word characteristics in general – something which is also supported by the established changes in the completely untrained skill areas. In this case, the systematic use of algorithmic and self-instructive methods in the skill areas selected could have had farther reaching, rather more unspecific transfer effects by having positively influenced not just the students' orthographic but the self-regulated and motivational competencies as well (Klauer, 2000). Corresponding improvements, e.g. with regard to the task-related attention required and the self-related competence and control cognitions, might in turn have had a reinforcing effect on the orthographic performances over time (Faber, 2002d; O'Mara, Marsh and Craven, 2004; Schunk, 1996). In this respect, more detailed results and findings can only be expected from suitable training studies which examine both specific and unspecific student performances as conditional variables.

CONCLUSION

The results of evaluation studies so far conducted in the field of systematic remedial training with graphic problem-solving algorithms and verbal self-instructions could establish and prove significant gains in performance on the part of four training cohorts whose intervention was completed after nearly two years in each case. In the meantime, the relevant analyses encompass an intervention period of about five years, and they are based on data compiled from overall N = 100 dyslexic children and adolescents (Figure 13) – not taking the ongoing study (with the fifth training cohort) into consideration.

Overall, it was possible to replicate and to gradually specify the pertinent results and findings:

- On the basis of relevant norm test scores, the students trained over a longer period of time were able, interindividually as well as intraindividually, to achieve highly significant gains in spelling performance. This result is maintained even when empirically taking into consideration regression-related gains in performance prior to the treatment.

- At the same time, the students trained over a longer period of time were able to achieve, particularly in statistical and practical terms, significant gains in the systematically trained spelling skill areas.

- To a slightly lesser but still significant extent, this also holds good for the spelling skill areas only incidentally considered. In this respect, strategic transfer effects must have taken place in the course of the intervention.

- The analyses could establish significant improvements in the untrained spelling skill areas as well, which also indicates the possibility of strategic transfer effects.

- The gains in performance achieved in each case and cohort were not significantly correlated to gender, age, or regular school training conditions.

- Finally, some first empirical evidences suggest that advances in the students' performance – with the proviso of conceptually adequate approaches, procedures, and training conditions – can be achieved largely independent of any teacher effects.

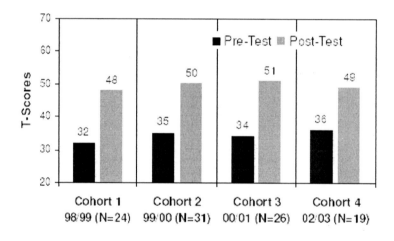

Figure 13. Spelling test performance in four training cohorts: Comparison of pre- and post-test data

Last but not least, the beneficial general conditions for the training have played an important role with regard to the extent of the performance gains achieved – above all, the continuous work in single or small group sessions as well as the extensive utilization of learning time available. On the basis of these preliminary results and findings, the efficiency of systematic remedial spelling training with problem-solving algorithms and self-instructions in the context of extracurricular educational activities, can hardly be disputed any longer. They seem to augment and specify the state of research in the evaluation of rule- and strategy-oriented interventions with severely dyslexic students – insofar as the results achieved by them repeatedly indicate the possibility of practically significant treatment effects in the conceptually trained spelling skill areas, as well as those incidentally considered and those not trained at all (Butyniec-Thomas and Woloshyn, 1997; Graham, Harris and Chorzempa, 2002; Lechner, 1985; Mäki, Vauras and Vainio, 2002; Mannhaupt, 2003; Matthes, 1994; Nock,

Sikorski and Thiel, 1988; Nunes, Bryant, and Olsson, 2003; Schulte-Körne, Deimel and Remschmidt, 1998, 2003; Tijms, Hoeks, Paulussen-Hoogeboom and Smolenaars, 2003; Walter, Bigga and Bischof, 1995; Wong, 1986).

These preliminary findings, however, have to be replicated again, by all means, with additional evaluation studies – and they have to be specified further with regard to a comprehensive series of conceptual and/or methodical questions of detail. Against the background of an extensive examination of the training process with respect to student personality and learning strategy, it still has to be clarified, inter alia,

- whether the single problem-solving algorithms and task formats had a differential effect on certain student groups, therefore possibly exerting a beneficial or adverse influence on their learning, depending upon existing behavioral and/or attention deficit problems to a variable extent (Murray, 1978; Reid, Trout and Schartz, 2005; Van Hell, Bosman and Bartelings, 2003),
- whether it is possible with this intervention approach to favorably change the students' academic self-perceptions, particularly their spelling-specific self-concept and their related test-anxious reactions, thus possibly reducing the cognitive-motivational blocks to their learning (Faber, 1991b, 1995, 2000, 2002e; O'Mara, Marsh and Craven, 2004; Schunk, 1986),
- and whether the combination of problem-solving algorithms, verbal self-instructions, and explicit strategy-specific feedback procedure can contribute to the development of conducive causal attributions for success and failure on the part of the students, thus reducing the individually perceived extent of spelling-specific helplessness on a long-term basis (Faber, 2002d; Clifford, 1990; Sideridis, 2003; Tabbassam and Grainger, 2003).

Independent from detailed conceptual perspectives of this nature, it might be interesting as well, eventually, to examine whether the visualizing and verbalizing methods developed can be systematically transferred to rule-specific spelling trainings in the orthographies of other languages, and whether they can be integrated into other training approaches phonologically oriented, and to conduct pertinent studies to this end (Berninger, Vaughan, Abbott, Brooks, Begay, Curtin, Byrd and Graham, 2000; Lovett, Lacerenza, Borden, Frijters, Steinbach and De Palma, 2000; Lyytinen, Aro and Holopainen, 2004; Tijms and Hoeks, 2005).

In this sense, it can be expected that further studies evaluating such interventions in practice will yield additional important findings as to the practicability and efficiency of the training using problem-solving algorithms and self-instructions – particularly when they are conducted on a long-term basis under everyday conditions, thus guaranteeing a high degree of ecological validity, and when their results can be used directly, if required, for didactical-methodical modifications in the concrete work with children and adolescents. They should be complemented in a timely manner with single-case analyses, particularly when individual difficulties are encountered in the course of the training, e.g. when students don not seem to benefit from the intervention to the extent expected (Faber, 2004c; Mäki, Vauras and Vainio, 2002).

Nevertheless, empirical analyses of this nature, accompanying the training in practice, can represent only one level of evaluation. For an adequate assessment, with regard to research methods, of intervention effects depending upon procedures and concepts in particular, it is essential to also conduct quasi-experimental field studies with relevant comparative data on untrained and/or alternatively trained student groups. Only the results of both types of empirical treatment evaluation allow extensively confirmed conclusions, sufficiently valid externally as well as internally, as to value and efficiency of the training approach presented.

REFERENCES

Arievitch, I.M. and Stetsenko, A. (2000). The quality of cultural tools and cognitive development: Gal'perin's perspective and its implications. *Human Development, 43*, 69-92.

Baird, J.R. and White, R.T. (1982). Promoting self-control of learning. *Instructional Science, 11*, 227-247.

Bailet, L.L. (1990). Spelling rule usage among students with learning disabilities and normally achieving students. *Journal of Learning Disabilities, 23*, 121-128.

Barkley, R.A. (1998). Attention deficit hyperactivity disorder – *A handbook for diagnosis and treatment* (2nd ed.). New York: Guilford.

Berninger, V.W., Vaughan, K., Abbott, R.D., Brooks, A., Begay, K., Curtin, G., Byrd, K. and Graham, S. (2000). Language-based spelling instruction: Teaching children to make multiple connections between spoken and written words. *Learning Disability Quarterly, 23*, 117-135.

Betz, D. and Breuninger, H. (1993). Teufelskreis Lernstörungen. *Theoretische Grundlegung und Standardprogramm* (3. Aufl.). Weinheim: Beltz.

Birkel, P. (1994a). Weingartener Grundwortschatz Rechtschreib-Test für zweite und dritte Klassen WRT 2+. Göttingen: Hogrefe.

Birkel, P. (1994b). Weingartener Grundwortschatz Rechtschreib-Test für dritte und vierte Klassen WRT 3+. Göttingen: Hogrefe.

Blachman, B.A., Schatschneider, C., Fletcher, J.M., Francis, D.J., Clonan, S.M., Shaywitz, B.A. and Shaywitz, S.E. (2004). Effects of intensive reading remediation for second and third graders and a 1-year follow-up. *Journal of Educational Psychology, 96*, 444-461.

Bodrova, E. and Leong, D.J. (1998). Scaffolding emergent writing in the zone of proximal development. *Literacy Teaching and Learning, 3*(2), 1-18.

Borkowski, J.G., Johnston, M.B. and Reid, M.K. (1987). Metacognition, motivation, and controlled performance. In S.J. Ceci (Ed.), *Handbook of cognitive, social, and neuropsychological aspects of learning disabilities.* Volume 2 (pp. 147-173). Hillsdale: Erlbaum.

Brown, A.L. and Campione, J.C. (1986). Psychological theory and the study of learning disabilities. *American Psychologist, 41*, 1059-1068.

Butyniec-Thomas, J. and Woloshyn, V.E. (1997). The effects of explicit-strategy and whole-language instruction on students' spelling ability. *Journal of Experimental Education, 65*, 293-302.

Carlisle, J. (1987). The use of morphological knowledge in spelling derived forms by LD and normal students. *Annals of Dyslexia, 37*, 90-108.

Carroll, J.M., Maughan, B., Goodman, R. and Meltzer, H. (2005). Literacy difficulties and psychiatric disorders: evidence for comorbidity. *Journal of Child Psychology and Psychiatry,* 46, 524-532.

Clarke, J.H. (1991). Using visual organizers to focus on thinking. *Journal of Reading,* 34, 526-534.

Clifford, M.M. (1990). Student motivation and academic achievement. In P. Vedder (Ed.), *Fundamental studies in educational research* (pp. 59-89). Lisse: Swets and Zeitlinger.

Cohen, J. (1986). Learning disabilities and psychological development in childhood and adolescence. *Annals of Dyslexia,* 36, 287-300.

Cohen, J. (1988). Statistical power analysis for the behavioral sciences (2nd ed.). Hillsdale: Erlbaum.

Darch, C.B. and Kame'enui, E.J. (2004). Instructional classroom management. *A proactive approach to behavior management* (2nd ed.). Upper Saddle River: Pearson Education.

Darch, C., Kim, S., Johnson, S. and James, H. (2000). The strategic spelling skills of students with learning disabilities: The results of two studies. *Journal of Instructional Psychology,* 27, 15-26.

Ellis, E.S., Deshler, D.D., Lens, B.K., Schumaker, J.B. and Clark, F.L. (1991). An instructional model for teaching learning strategies. *Focus on Exceptional Children,* 23(6), 1-24.

Faber, G. (1991a). Lehrerkompetenzen zur Entwicklung schülerzentrierter Arbeitsformen in der Rechtschreibförderung. In H. Knopf (Hrsg.), Psychologie in der Lehrerbildung (S. 136-146). Martin-Luther-Universität Halle-Wittenberg: *Wissenschaftsbereich Psychologie.*

Faber, G. (1991b). Entwicklung und Erprobung eines Fragebogens zum rechtschreibbezogenen Selbstkonzept von Grundschülern. *Empirische Pädagogik,* 5, 317-347.

Faber, G. (1995). Die Diagnose von Leistungsangst vor schulischen Rechtschreibsituationen: Neue Ergebnisse zu den psychometrischen Kennwerten und zur Validität einer entsprechenden Kurzskala. *Praxis der Kinderpsychologie und Kinderpsychiatrie,* 44, 110-119.

Faber, G. (2000). Rechtschreibängstliche Besorgtheits- und Aufgeregtheitskognitionen: Empirische Untersuchungsergebnisse zum subjektiven Kompetenz- und Bedrohungserleben rechtschreibschwacher Grundschulkinder. *Sonderpädagogik,* 30, 191-201.

Faber, G. (2001a). Visualisierte Lösungsalgorithmen in der Arbeit mit rechtschreibschwachen Schulkindern: Ein Ansatz zum systematischen Aufbau orthographischer Regelkenntnisse und Handlungsstrategien. *Sonderpädagogik,* 31, 108-117.

Faber, G. (2001b). Materialien zur Förderung orthographischer Kompetenzen. Band 1: Visualisierte Lösungsalgorithmen und verbale Selbstinstruktionen im Lernbereich gk. Goslar: Brumby.

Faber, G. (2002a). Materialien zur Förderung orthographischer Kompetenzen. Band 2: Visualisierte Lösungsalgorithmen und verbale Selbstinstruktionen im Lernbereich dt. Goslar: Brumby.

Faber, G. (2002b). Materialien zur Förderung orthographischer Kompetenzen. Band 3: Visualisierte Lösungsalgorithmen und verbale Selbstinstruktionen im Lernbereich ie. Goslar: Brumby.

Faber, G. (2002c). Algorithmische und selbstinstruktive Lernhilfen in der Rechtschreibförderung. Konzept und Anwendung visualisierter Lösungspläne. *Zeitschrift für Heilpädagogik,* 53, 194–198.

Faber, G. (2002d). Diktatbezogene Erfolgs- und Misserfolgsattributionen: Empirische Untersuchungsergebnisse zum subjektiven Kompetenz- und Kontrollerleben rechtschreibschwacher Grundschulkinder. *Heilpädagogische Forschung,* 28, 2-10.

Faber, G. (2002e). Rechtschreibängstliche Besorgtheits- und Aufgeregtheitskognitionen: Empirische Untersuchungsergebnisse zu ihrer Bedeutung für das Selbstwertgefühl und die Schulunlust rechtschreibschwacher Grundschulkinder. *Sonderpädagogik,* 32, 3-12.

Faber, G. (2003a). Materialien zur Förderung orthographischer Kompetenzen. Band 4: Visualisierte Lösungsalgorithmen und verbale Selbstinstruktionen im Lernbereich II. Goslar: Brumby.

Faber, G. (2003b). Der systematische Einsatz visualisierter Lösungsalgorithmen und verbaler Selbstinstruktionen in der Rechtschreibförderung: Erste Ergebnisse praxisbegleitender Effektkontrollen. *Praxis der Kinderpsychologie und Kinderpsychiatrie,* 52, 677-688.

Faber, G. (2003c). Lösungsalgorithmen und Selbstinstruktionen in der Rechtschreibförderung. *Kindheit und Entwicklung,* 12, 243–248.

Faber, G. (2003d). Lese-Rechtschreibprobleme: Explorativer Fragebogen für Eltern. Vorläufige Arbeitsversion (pdf-Datei auf CD-ROM). Goslar: *Arbeitsstelle für pädagogische Entwicklung und Förderung.*

Faber, G. (2004a). Stimmlos, lang… also mit ß! – Systematische Rechtschreibförderung mit algorithmischen Lösungsplänen und Aufgabenformaten im Lernbereich s-Laute. *Materialien für den Klassen- und Förderunterricht.* Clausthal-Zellerfeld: Papierflieger.

Faber, G. (2004b). Allgemeine und spezifische Veränderungen in den orthographischen Kompetenzen rechtschreibschwacher Schüler: Die Ergebnisse praxisbegleitender Effektkontrollen nach einer zweijährigen Förderung mit algorithmischen und selbstinstruktiven Lernhilfen. *Sonderpädagogik,* 34, 150–164.

Faber, G. (2004c). Algorithmische und selbstinstruktive Lernhilfen in der Rechtschreibförderung. Exemplarische Einzelfallanalysen zur systematischen Entwicklung orthographischer Schülerkompetenzen. *Zeitschrift für Heilpädagogik,* 55, 487–496.

Faber, G. (2004d). Lernhilfen. Kopiervorlagen zur systematischen Rechtschreibförderung: 45 kommentierte Arbeitsblätter auf CD-ROM (pdf-Datei). Goslar: Arbeitsstelle für pädagogische Entwicklung und Förderung.

Faber, G. (2005a). Denkwörter – Schülerheft 7. Vertiefende Übungen zur lernstrategischen Sicherung orthographischer Kompetenzen im Lernbereich gk+ (gk, dt, bp, sz und h). Goslar: Arbeitsstelle für pädagogische Entwicklung und Förderung.

Faber, G. (2005b). Sprechwörter – Schülerheft 15. Vertiefende Übungen zur lernstrategischen Sicherung lautsprachlicher und alphabetischer Kompetenzen im Lernbereich bd. Goslar: Arbeitsstelle für pädagogische Entwicklung und Förderung.

Faber, G. (2005c). Die Arbeit mit visualisierten Lösungsalgorithmen und verbalen Selbstinstruktionen in der Rechtschreibförderung – exemplarische Darstellung einer methodischen Möglichkeit. *Die Sprachheilarbeit,* 50, 176-181.

Faber, G. (2005d). Förderung orthographischer Schülerkompetenzen durch die systematische Verwendung algorithmischer und selbstinstruktiver Lernhilfen: Empirische Befunde zu den vorläufigen Veränderungen in ausgewählt trainierten und untrainierten Rechtschreibbereichen. *Sonderpädagogik,* 35 (in press).

Frith, U. (1985). Beneath the surface of developmental dyslexia. In K.E. Patterson, J.C. Marshall and M. Coltheart (Eds.), Surface dyslexia. Neuropsychological and cognitive studies of phonological reading (pp. 301-330). Hillsdale: Erlbaum.

Gal'perin, P.Ya. (1989a). Mental actions as a basis for the formation of thoughts and images. *Soviet Psychology,* 27(3), 45-64.

Gal'perin, P.Ya. (1989b). Organization of mental activity and the effectiveness of learning. *Soviet Psychology,* 27(3), 65-82.

Gal'perin, P.Ya. (1989c). The problem of attention. *Soviet Psychology,* 27(3), 83-92.

Graham, S., Harris, K.R. and Chorzempa, B.F. (2002). Contribution of spelling instruction to the spelling, writing, and reading of poor spellers. *Journal of Educational Psychology,* 94, 669-686.

Grund, M., Haug, G. *and* Naumann, C.L. (1994). DRT 4. Diagnostischer Rechtschreibtest für 4. Klassen. Weinheim: Beltz.

Grund, M., Haug, G. *and* Naumann, C.L. (1995). DRT 5. Diagnostischer Rechtschreibtest für 5. Klassen. Weinheim: Beltz.

Harris, K.R. (1990). Developing self-regulated learners: The role of private speech and self-instructions. *Educational Psychologist,* 25, 35-49.

Heiervang, E., Stevenson, J., Lund, A. and Hugdahl, K. (2001). Behaviour problems in children with dyslexia. *Nordic Journal of Psychiatry,* 55, 251-256.

Humphrey, N. (2003). Facilitating a positive sense of self in pupils with dyslexia: the role of teachers and peers. *Support for Learning,* 18(3), 130-136.

Humphrey, N. and Mullins, P.M. (2002). Personal constructs and attribution for academic success and failure in dyslexia. *British Journal of Special Education,* 29, 196-203.

Klauer, K.J. (2000). Das Huckepack-Theorem asymmetrischen Strategietransfers. Ein Beitrag zur Trainings- und Transfertheorie. *Zeitschrift für Entwicklungspsychologie und Pädagogische Psychologie,* 32, 153-165.

Klauer, K.J. and Lauth, G.W. (1997). Lernbehinderungen und Leistungsschwierigkeiten bei Schülern. In F.E. Weinert (Hrsg.), Psychologie des Unterrichts und der Schule. *Enzyklopädie der Psychologie: Pädagogische Psychologie* 3 (S. 701-738). Göttingen: Hogrefe.

Klicpera, C. and Gasteiger-Klicpera, B. (1995). Psychologie der Lese-Rechtschreibschwierigkeiten. Entwicklung, Ursachen, Förderung. Weinheim: Beltz.

Klicpera, C. and Schabmann, A. (1993). Do German-speaking children have a chance to overcome reading and spelling difficulties? A longitudinal survey from the second until the eighth grade. *European Journal of Psychology of Education,* 8, 307-323

Kossow, H.-J. (1979). Zur Therapie der Lese-Rechtschreibschwäche. Aufbau und Erprobung eines theoretisch begründeten Therapieprogramms (6. Aufl.). Berlin: Deutscher Verlag der Wissenschaften.

Landerl, K. (2003). Categorization of vowel length in German poor spellers: An orthographically relevant phonological distinction. *Applied Psycholinguistics,* 24, 523-538.

Larkin, M.J. *and* Ellis, E.S. (2004). Strategic academic interventions for adolescents with learning disabilities. In B.Y.L. Wong (Ed.), *Learning about learning disabilities* (3rd ed., pp 375-414). San Diego: Elsevier.

Lechner, A. (1985). Trainingsprogramm zur schulrelevanten Aufmerksamkeit im Unterrichtsfach Deutsch. Universität Wien, Grund- und Integrativwissenschaftliche Fakultät: unveröffentlichte Dissertation.

Licht, B.G. *and* Kistner, J.A. (1986). Motivational problems of learning-disabled children: Individual differences and their implications for treatment. In J.K. Torgensen *and* B.Y.L. Wong (Eds.), Psychological and educational perspectives on learning disabilities (pp. 225-255). Orlando: Academic Press.

Lovett, M.W., Lacerenza, L., Borden, S.L., Frijters, J.C., Steinbach, K.A. *and* De Palma, M. (2000). Components of effective remediation for developmental reading disabilities: Combining phonological and strategy-based instruction to improve outcomes. *Journal of Educational Psychology, 92*, 263-283.

Lyytinen, H., Aro, M. *and* Holopainen, L. (2004). Dyslexia in highly orthographically regular Finnish. In I. Smythe, J. Everatt *and* R. Salter (Eds.), International book of dyslexia. A cross-language comparison and practice guide (pp. 81-91). Chichester: Wiley.

Mäki, H.S., Vauras, M.M.S. *and* Vainio, S. (2002). Reflective spelling strategies for elementary school students with severe writing difficulties: A case study. Learning Disability Quarterly, 25, 189-207.

Manis, F.R. *and* Morrison, F.J. (1985). Reading disability: A deficit in rule learning. In L.S. Siegel *and* F.J. Morrison (Eds.), Cognitive development in atypical children (pp. 1-26). New York: Springer.

Mann, C. (1991). Selbstbestimmtes Rechtschreiblernen. Rechtschreibunterricht als Strategievermittlung. Weinheim: Beltz.

Mannhaupt, G. (1999). Strategische und entwicklungsorientierte Fördermaßnahmen im Rechtschreiben. Kindheit und Entwicklung, 8, 158–161.

Mannhaupt, G. (2003). Ergebnisse von Therapiestudien. In W. von Suchodoletz (Hrsg.), Therapie der Lese-Rechtschreib-Störung (LRS). Traditionelle und alternative Behandlungsmethoden im Überblick (S. 91-107). Stuttgart: Kohlhammer.

Masendorf, F. (1997). Einführung in das Experiment im Kontext sonderpädagogischer Theoriebildung. In F. Masendorf (Hrsg.), Experimentelle Sonderpädagogik. Ein Lehrbuch zur angewandten Forschung (S. 71-75). Weinheim: Beltz.

Matthes, G. (1994). Vermittlung positiver Lernerfahrungen bei extremen Rechtschreibschwierigkeiten. *Heilpädagogische Forschung, 20*, 56-65.

May, P. (1998). HSP 5–9. Hamburger Schreibprobe für die Klassen 5 bis 9. Hamburg: Verlag für pädagogische Medien.

Meichenbaum, D. and Asarnow, J. (1979). Cognitive-behavioral modification and metacognitive development: Implications for the classroom. In P.C. Kendall and S.D. Hollon (Eds.), Cognitive-behavioral interventions. *Theory, research, and practice* (pp. 11-35). New York: Academic Press.

Miller, G.E. and Brewster, M.E. (1992). Developing self-sufficient learners in reading and mathematics through self-instructional training. In M. Pressley, K.R. Harris and J.T. Guthrie (Eds.), Promoting academic competence and literacy in schools (pp. 169-222). San Diego: Academic Press.

Montague, M. (1997). Cognitive strategy instruction in mathematics for students with learning disabilities. *Journal of Learning Disabilities, 30*, 164-177.

Murray, M.E. (1978). The relationship between personality adjustment and success in remedial programs for dyslexic children. *Contemporary Educational Psychology, 3*, 330-339.

Nock, H., Sikorski, P.B. and Thiel, R.-D. (1988). Die Veränderung der Rechtschreibleistung durch Selbststeuerung des Denkens in der Diktatsituation. Untersuchungsbericht zu den Auswirkungen gezielter psychologisch-pädagogischer Zusatzmaßnahmen zur Veränderung des Denkens bei Realschülern der Klassenstufe 5. Lehren und Lernen, 14(3), 1-63.

Nolen-Hoeksema, S., Girgus, J.S. and Seligman, M.E.P. (1986). Learned helplessness in children: A longitudinal study of depression, achievement, and explanatory style. *Journal of Personality and Social Psychology, 51*, 435-442.

Nunes, T., Bryant, P. and Olsson, J. (2003). Learning morphological and phonological spelling rules: An intervention study. *Scientific Studies of Reading, 7*, 289-307.

O'Mara, A.J., Marsh, H.W. and Craven, R.G. (2004). Self-concept enhancement: A meta-analysis integrating a multidimensional perspective. Paper presented at the Third International Biennial SELF Research Conference: Self-concept, motivation and identity. Where to from here? Berlin: Max Planck Institute for Human Development [http://self.uws.edu.au/Conferences/2004_O'Mara_Marsh_Craven.pdf].

Peers, I.S. (1996). Statistical analysis for education and psychology researchers. London: Falmer Press.

Poskiparta, E., Niemi, P., Lepola, J., Ahtola, A. and Laine, P. (2003). Motivational-emotional vulnerability and difficulties in learning to read and spell. *British Journal of Educational Psychology, 73*, 187-206.

Pressley, M. (1986). The relevance of the good strategy user model to the teaching of mathematics. *Educational Psychologist, 21*, 139-161.

Reid, D.K. (1988). Learning and learning to learn. In D.K. Reid (Ed.), Teaching the learning disabled. *A cognitive developmental approach* (pp. 5-28). Boston: Allyn and Bacon.

Reid, R., Trout, A.L. and Schartz, M. (2005). Self-regulation interventions for children with attention deficit/hyperactivity disorder. *Exceptional Children, 71*, 361-377.

Rieder, O. (1984). Rechtschreibtest für 6. und 7. Klassen RST 6-7. Weinheim: Beltz.

Röber-Siekmeyer, C. (1993). Die Schriftsprache entdecken. Rechtschreiben im offenen Unterricht. Weinheim: Beltz.

Rogosa, D.R. *and* Willett, J.B. (1985). Understanding correlates of change by modeling individual differences in growth. *Psychometrika, 50*, 203-228.

Scheerer-Neumann, G. (1979). Intervention bei Lese-Rechtschreibschwäche. Überblick über Themen, Methoden und Ergebnisse. Bochum: Kamp.

Scheerer-Neumann, G. (1988). Rechtschreibtraining mit rechtschreibschwachen Hauptschülern auf kognitionspsychologischer Grundlage: Eine empirische Untersuchung. Opladen: Westdeutscher Verlag.

Scheerer-Neumann, G. (1993). Interventions in developmental reading and spelling disorders. In H. Grimm and H. Skowronek (Eds.), Language acquisition problems and reading disorders: Aspects of diagnosis and intervention (pp. 319-352). Berlin: de Gruyter.

Schulte-Körne, G., Deimel, W. and Remschmidt, H. (1998). Das Marburger Eltern-Kind-Rechtschreibtraining – Verlaufsuntersuchung nach zwei Jahren. Zeitschrift für Kinder- und Jugendpsychiatrie, 26, 167-173.

Schulte-Körne, G., Deimel, W. and Remschmidt. H. (2003). Rechtschreibtraining in schulischen Fördergruppen – Ergebnisse einer Evaluationsstudie in der Primarstufe. Zeitschrift für Kinder- und Jugendpsychiatrie und Psychotherapie, 31, 85-98.

Schulte-Körne, G. *and* Mathwig, F. (2001). Das Marburger Rechtschreibtraining. Ein regelgeleitetes Förderprogramm für rechtschreibschwache Kinder. Bochum: Winkler.

Schunk, D.H. (1986). Verbalization and children's self-regulated learning. *Contemporary Educational Psychology,* 11, 347-369.

Schunk, D.H. and Rice, J.M. (1987). Enhancing comprehension skill and self-efficacy with strategy value information. *Journal of Reading Behavior,* 19, 285-302.

Scott, K.S. (1999). Cognitive instructional strategies. In W.N. Bender (Ed.), Professional issues in learning disabilities. *Practical strategies and relevant research findings* (pp. 55-82). Austin: Pro-Ed.

Sideridis, G.D. (2003). On the origins of helpless behaviour of students with learning disabilities: avoidance motivation? *International Journal of Educational Research,* 39, 497-517.

Steffler, D.J. (2004). An investigation of Grade 5 children's knowledge of the doubling rule in spelling. *Journal of Research in Reading,* 27, 248-264.

Stolla, G. (2000). Bausteine für ein erfolgreiches Lernen und Üben im Rechtschreiben. Teil 2: Weitere Grundlagen und erste Einsichten. Heinsberg: Dieck.

Tabassam, W. and Grainger, J. (2003). Self-concept enhancement for students with learning difficulties with and without attention deficit hyperactivity disorder. In H.W. Marsh, R.G. Craven and D.M. McInerney (Eds.), *International advances in self research* (pp. 231-260). Greenwich: Information Age Publishing.

Tacke, G., Wörner, R., Schultheiß, G. and Brezing, H. (1993). Die Auswirkung rhythmisch-syllabierenden Mitsprechens auf die Rechtschreibleistung. Zeitschrift für Pädagogische Psychologie, 7, 139-147.

Thackwray, D., Meyers, A., Schleser, R. and Cohen, R. (1985). Achieving generalization with general versus specific self-instructions: Effects on academically deficient children. *Cognitive Therapy and Research,* 9, 297-308.

Tijms, J. and Hoeks, J. (2005). A computerized treatment of dyslexia: Benefits from treating lexico-phonological processing problems. *Dyslexia,* 11, 22-40.

Tijms, J., Hoeks, J.J.W.M., Paulussen-Hoogeboom, M.C. and Smolenaars, A.J. (2003). Long-term effects of a psycholinguistic treatment for dyslexia. *Journal of Research in Reading,* 26, 121-140.

Tobias, S. (1992). The impact of test anxiety on cognition in school learning. In K.A. Hagtvet and T.B. Johnson (Eds.), *Advances in test anxiety research.* Volume 7 (pp. 18-31). Lisse: Swets and Zeitlinger.

Topping, K.J. (1995). Cued spelling: A powerful technique for parent and peer tutoring. *The Reading Teacher,* 48, 374-383.

Valtin, R., Badel, I., Löffler, I., Meyer-Schepers, U. and Voss, A. (2003). Orthographische Kompetenzen von Schülerinnen und Schülern der vierten Klasse. In W. Bos, E.-M. Lankes, M. Prenzel, K. Schwippert, G. Walther and R. Valtin (Hrsg.), Erste Ergebnisse aus IGLU. Schülerleistungen am Ende der vierten Jahrgangsstufe im internationalen Vergleich (S. 227-264). Münster: Waxmann.

Van Hell, J.G., Bosman, A.M.T. and Bartelings, M.C.G. (2003). Visual dictation improves the spelling performance of three groups of Dutch students with spelling disabilities. *Learning Disability Quarterly,* 26, 239-255.

Walter, J., Bigga, R. and Bischof, H. (1995). Computergestützte Intervention bei Rechtschreibschwäche: Effekte eines kognitions- und lernpsychologisch orientierten Trainingsprogramms auf Morphembasis. *Sonderpädagogik,* 25, 4-22.

Weber, J.-M., Marx, P. and Schneider, W. (2002). Profitieren Legastheniker und allgemein lese-rechtschreibschwache Kinder in unterschiedlichem Ausmaß von einem Rechtschreibtraining? *Psychologie in Erziehung und Unterricht,* 49, 56-70.

Weigt, R. (1994). Lesen- und Schreibenlernen kann jeder!? Methodische Hilfen bei Lese-Rechtschreibschwäche. Neuwied: Luchterhand.

Wong, B.Y.L. (1986). A cognitive approach to teaching spelling. *Exceptional Children,* 53, 169-173.

Zutell, J. (1996). The Directed Spelling Thinking Activity (DSTA): Providing an effective balance in word study instruction. *The Reading Teacher,* 50, 98-108.

In: Dyslexia in Children: New Research
Editor: Christopher B. Hayes, pp. 47-64

ISBN 1-59454-969-9

Chapter 2

AUDIO-VISUAL TRAINING IN THE DISCRIMINATION OF THE PHONETIC FEATURE OF VOICING IN DYSLEXIC CHILDREN

Annie Magnan[1], Jean Ecalle[1], and Jean-Emile Gombert[2]
[1] Laboratoire d'Etude des Mécanismes Cognitifs/Laboratoire Dynamique du Langage
UMR-CNRS 5596 Université Lumière Lyon 2 - France
[2] Centre de Recherche en Psychologie, Cognition et Communication
Université Rennes 2 - France

ABSTRACT

Dyslexic children are characterized by a phoneme awareness deficit and the associated problems in performing decoding. In particular, most reading errors are due to confusions between phonemes which differ on minimal traits (especially voiced-unvoiced oppositions). Dyslexics may have a poorer categorical perception of certain contrasts.

In this study, we hypothesize that specific audio-visual training which aids phonetic feature perception could help dyslexic children to specify phonemic representations. Consequently, they should not confuse close phonemes on the phonetic features which could facilitate written word processing. Our aim was to test the effectiveness of an audio-visual training program designed to improve the discrimination of the phonetic feature of voicing on dyslexic children's recognition of written words.

Sixteen dyslexic children were separated into two equal groups strictly matched on educational and cognitive levels, as well as on reading level which was assessed using a standardized word reading test. The children in the experimental group received the audio-visual training whereas the children in the control group used a computerized "talking book" program. This system program enabled the children to read sentences on the computer under whole word and syllable feedback conditions. The reading material consisted of a set of stories selected from children's literature. The experimental training focused on paired-item voicing oppositions and involved six pairs of phonemes: /p/-/b/; /t/-/d/; /k/-/g/; /f/-/v/; /s/-/z/ and /ch/-/j/.

A traditional pre-test, interventiontraining phase, and post-test design was used. Tests included a word recognition test and reading comprehension were tested. The results show the impact of audio-visual training on the performances of the dyslexic children in the word reading task. It proved possible to improve phonological representations by means of training which involved both phonological and orthographic units. The effectiveness of this audio-visual training is discussed both in the light of the phonetic model - the phonological deficits in dyslexic children may be partly due to impairments in the phonetic organization of phoneme detectors, as well as in terms of a connectionist model of reading development (Harm &and Seidenberg, 1999).

DYSLEXIA: WHAT ARE THE CAUSES?

Developmental dyslexia is defined as a difficulty in reading and spellinglearning to read despite the presence of the intelligence, motivation, and education necessary for successful reading and in the absence of any obvious neurological or sensory disorders. Studies have shown that the reading deficits of children with developmental dyslexia persist into adolescence and even adulthood. Its prevalence is still actively being examined but has been estimated at at any where betweenapproximately 5 and 10% of the population. It therefore represents a very significant national and international concern (Shaywitz, 1998).

The exact cause of dyslexia is still unknown. However, researchers believe agree that dyslexia is a reading disability with underlying genetic, developmental and neurological causes (Frith, 1997). In Frith's well-known account, dyslexia is seen as a cultural phenomenon that also has cognitive and biological bases. Today, the fundamental causes of dyslexia are actively being researched (Temple, 2002; Ramus 2001; 2003).

A consensus among many researchers is that developmental dyslexia is characterized by difficulties in phonological processing, and more specifically phonological awareness which is the ability to identify and manipulate the sound structure of words (Fawcett, 2001; Hulme &and Snowling, 1997; Snowling, 2000). Individuals with dyslexia have impaired phonological skills, including the ability to distinguish rhyming sounds, count the syllables of words, and identify novel or "pseudo-words" (e.g., "stroat" or "train"). Phonological awareness is a good predictor of early learning reading ability (Bradley &and Bryant, 1983; Mann, 1984; Shankweiler &and Liberman, 1989; see also Castles &and Coltheart, 2004 and Morais, 2003, for recent reviews). Impairments to phonological representation are implicated in at leastmost (ifth not all) some formscases of developmental dyslexia (Manis, Seidenberg, Doi, MacBride-Chang, &and Peterson, 1996 ; Stanovich, Siegel, &and Gottardo, 1997).

The phonological theory of dyslexia argues that dyslexics have impaired reading abilities because of a deficit in phonological processing. These phonological difficulties manifest themselves in different tasks including tests of phonological awareness, rapid automatic naming, verbal short-term memory, and speech perception (Stanovich &and Siegel, 1994; Torgesen, 1999). Because reading acquisition requires the child to learn the mapping between orthography and phonology (Jorm, Share, MacLean, &and Matthews, 1984; Share, 1995), problems in the representation and use of phonological information inevitably lead to problems in reading acquisition (Bradley &and Bryant, 1983; Bryant &and Bradley, 1985; Goswami &and Bryant, 1990). According to this model, dyslexics encounter difficulties with written language because they have an impaired ability to analyze written words into phonemes, thus preventing word identification (Goswami, 2000). This low-level phonological deficit prevents words from acceding to high-level linguistic processing which would allow the reader to gain meaning from the text. Thus, dyslexics have intact memory and language comprehension processes that remain unactivated because they can only be activated after a word has been identified through phonological processing (Frith 1997, Snowling, 2000).

The underlying cause of phonological deficits in dyslexic children is unclear although many different theories have attempted to account for these disorders. One approach suggests that dyslexia arises from deficits in systems that are specifically linguistic (also known as the domain-specific view). Dyslexia, in this view, arises from deficits in phonological memory and processing, i.e. processes specific to speech sounds (Snowling, 1998). A more basic auditory processing deficit has also been considered as a possible underlying cause of speech perception problems and the phonological deficit (Farmer &and Klein, 1995; Tallal, 1980). The auditory processing hypothesis suggests that auditory deficits are responsible for the phonological deficits are due to the auditory deficits, which in turn lead to the language disorder. Support for this hypothesis has been provided by evidence that dyslexics achieve poor performances in various auditory tasks including frequency discrimination (Mac Anally &and Stein, 1996; Ahissar, Protopapas, Reid, &and Merzenich, 2000) and temporal order judgment (Tallal 1980; Nagarajan, Mahncke, Salz, Tallal, Roberts, &and Merzenich, 1999). A deficit in representing short sounds and fast transitions would cause difficulties when such acoustic events are the cues for phonemic contrasts as in /ba/ versus /da/ (Adlard &and Hazan, 1998; Blomert &and Mitterer, 2004; Mody, Studdert-Kennedy, &and Brady, 1997; Rosen &and Manganari, 2001; Serniclaes, Sprenger-Charolles, Carré, &and Démonet, 2001; Serniclaes, Van Heghe, Mousty, Carré, &and Sprenger-Charolles, 2004). However, some studies of individual results have suggested that only a minority of dyslexics (40 to 50%) have speech categorization problems (Ramus, Rosen, Dakin, Day, Castellote, &and White, 2003; Rosen &and Manganari, 2001; Share, Jorm, MacLean, &and Matthews, 2002). Thus, the majority of dyslexics do not exhibit any auditory problems. There is no evidence that phonological difficulties stem from impairments of rapid auditory processing (Marshall, Snowling, &and Bailey, 2001). A recent review of the literature (Rosen, 2003) reveals suggests that some, but not all, auditory skills are impaired, on average, in groups of SLI and dyslexic listeners. Typically, only a minority of SLI and dyslexic listeners exhibit any auditory deficits, and there is little or no relationship between the severity of the auditory and language deficits in SLI and dyslexic groups. Indeed, this type of relationship is sometimes found to be stronger in control groups. Rosen suggests that auditory deficits do not appear to be causally related to language disorders, but simply occur in association with them.

TWell, this hypothesis of a deficit in categorical perception has led to the development and application of a computerized remediation program which has achieved good results in alleviating SLI, primarily by improving auditory processing (Merzenich, Jenkins, Johnston, Schreiner, Miller, &and Tallal 1996; Tallal, Miller, Bedi, Byma, Wang, Nagarajan, et al., 1996). These authors have reported success in directly modifying children's ability to process the rapidly changing features of auditory signals or signal features which occur in rapid succession.

However, negative results have also been reported in connection with this method and the associated theory (Mody, Studdert-Kennedy, &and Brady, 1997; Nittrouer, 1999). Consequently its value as a widely used technique for aiding children with reading disabilities is still uncertain.

To summarize, the two leading current hypotheses concerning the information processing weaknesses that result in performance difficulties on the two key measures, namely phonological awareness and alphabetic reading skills, are a speech-specific perceptual processing problem (Studdert-Kennedy &and Mody, 1995) on the one hand, and, on the other, a more general problem in the processing of rapidly changing acoustic stimuli or stimuli that occur in rapid succession (Tallal, 1980).

Several theoretical accounts of dyslexia cite a fundamental deficit in the processing and representation of phonological information (Harm &and Seidenberg, 1999; Manis, Seidenberg, Doi, McBrideChang, &and Petersen, 1996; Rayner, Foorman, Perfetti, Pesetsky, &and Seidenberg, 2001; Share, 1995; Stanovich &and Siegel, 1994) which is due to a flawed analysis of the sound structure of words and/or inaccurate phonological representations of words (Swan &and Goswami, 1997). Harm and Seidenberg (1999) simulated phonological dyslexia in a connectionist model by introducing anomalies in phonological processing that were severe enough to affect reading acquisition but not the categorical perception of phonemes. Thus, the model suggests that phonological impairments can have causes other than a speech perception impairment and predicts that at least some phonological dyslexics will have normal speech perception.

Today, there is much evidence that dyslexics' reading can be substantially improved through intensive individualized instruction that focuses both on phonological skills and accurate reading in context.

COMPUTER-ASSISTED PROGRAMS FOR DYSLEXIC CHILDREN

Many studies of computer software have shown its potential to enhance phonological awareness in pre-school children (Chera &and Wood, 2003; Hecht &and Close, 2002), in mainstream school children (Moore, Rosenberg, &and Coleman, 2005), and in children with reading difficulties (Magnan &and Ecalle, in press). Computer-based reading instruction is a relatively new and promising approach for the teaching of phonemic awareness (Torgersen &and Barker, 1995). Computer-aided learning is often promoted as offering a flexible environment. The qualities of computers that are relevant to instruction in phonemic awareness include digitized speech and high-quality graphics, immediate feedback and a game-like presentation which keeps children interested (Mioduser, Tur-Kaspa, &and Leitner, 2000).

An important factor in the development of computer technology for reading instruction has been the availability of high-quality text-to-speech translation. Olson, Foltz, and Wise, (1986), Olson and Wise, (1992), Wise, Ring, and Olson (2000) have explored the use of synthetic computer speech as a remedial tool for dyslexic children's deficits in printed word recognition. In their initial studies, these authors selected children in 3rd to 6th grade who were in the lower 10% of their classes in reading. The children read stories on the computer for a half an hour each day. When they encountered difficult words in the stories, they could click on the words with a mouse to make the computer highlight and pronounce the words. During the session, the children answered occasional multiple-choice comprehension questions about the stories they were reading on the computer. At the end of the session, the computer presented some of the targeted words in a recognition test. The average word-reading gains of the computer-trained children significantly exceeded those of matched poor readers who remained in their regular reading class. However, some of the computer-trained children had difficulty working alone with the programs. Olson and Wise (1992) found that the children's phonological skills at the start of training were positively correlated with their rate of word-reading improvement during training, thus suggesting that directly remediating such children's phonological-processing deficits might make a useful contribution to their reading development. The benefits of different kinds of speech segmentation (whole word, syllables, onset-rimes and phoneme segmentation) were compared. Subsequently, Olson, Wise, Ring and Johnson (1997) used a different program and training environment to conducted a longitudinal study. They trained children with reading problems attending 2nd to 5th grade in small groups of 3 or 4 children, each with their own computer and with a teacher always present. The programs included reading stories on the computer with help for difficult words, as in the authors' previous studies. In addition, half of the children spent part of their training time working with programs designed to improve their deficient phoneme awareness and phonological decoding skills. The other children spent all their time accurately reading stories and applying strategies for understanding and remembering the stories. The phonological training programs were very effective in improving children's phonological skills, and this improvement was associated with significantly greater gains in several word-reading tests performed by the youngest and worst readers. However, the older and more skilled poor readers in the 4th and 5th grades seemed to gain as much or more in terms of word reading measures if they spent all their time accurately reading the stories on the computer and practicing their comprehension strategies (Wise, Ring, &and Olson, 1999; Wise et al., 2000). Olofsson (1992) developed a similar computer program using a Scandinavian text-to-speech unit which allowed children to read a text on the screen and use the mouse to request the pronunciation of a word. Others researchers have created a similar system and investigated different types of feed-back (Van Daal &and Reitsma, 1990; Elbro, Ramussen &and Spelling, 1996).

To summarize, the existing literature shows that segmented speech feedback is often effective in increasing phonological awareness (Olson et al., 1997; Van Daal, Reitsma, Van Der Leig, 1994). These studies have compared children who have been exposed to different forms of speech segmentation (whole word feedback or segmented word (onset-rime) feedback). The most common method of training phonological skills (Mitchell &and Fox, 2001; Wise et al., 1999) involves different sub-lexical units such as rime, syllable or phoneme. However, the results of research which attempt to train children's phonological awareness skills in order to improve their reading ability are mixed. Some computer-based interventions have not been very successful. For instance, Olson et al. (1997) and Wise and Olson (1995) have both reported improved phonological awareness but poor results in word recognition.

The impact of phonological awareness training on phonological awareness and reading skills has been examined in two quantitative meta-analyses (Bus &and Ijzendoorn, 1999; Ehri, Nunes, Stahl, &and Willows, 2001). These have demonstrated that speech-only approaches are minimally effective at impacting reading abilities. The results of the meta-analysis conducted by Ehri et al. (2001) showed that the scale of the reading improvement obtained using phonological awareness training with letters was roughly twice that obtained using similar speech-only activities.

According to connectionist models (Harm &and Seidenberg, 1999; Seidenberg &and McClelland, 1989), although some initial orthographic and phonological connections may be "taught" explicitly, the majority of such learning occurs through coincidence detection of probabilistic properties in the input, and is thus implicit. It is possible that orthography-to-meaning computations also involve implicit learning (Harm &and Seidenberg, 2004).

McCandliss, Beck, Sandak, and Perfetti (2003) examined the reading skills of children with deficient decoding skills in the years following the first grade, and traced their progress over 20 sessions of a decoding skills intervention program called Word Building developed by Beck (Beck, 1989; Beck &and Hamilton, 2000). At the start of the program, the children exhibited deficits in decoding, reading comprehension and phonemic awareness skills. The intervention directed attention to each grapheme position within a word by means of a procedure involving the *progressive minimal pairing* of words that differed by one grapheme. This activity provides a set of words that differ by a single grapheme. A child forms the words with letter cards by stepping through a scripted set of transformations that change one word into the next by changing a single grapheme at the beginning, middle, or end of the word. After each transformation, the child decodes the new word, which looks and sounds similar to the previously decoded word. This activity focuses attention on each individual letter sound unit within words and may play an important role in developing fully-specified representations of printed words. Harm, MacCandliss and Seidenberg (2003) have used the connectionist model of reading development, which is intended to simulate detailed aspects of developmental dyslexia (Harm &and Seidenberg, 1999), to examine why certain types of interventions designed to overcome reading impairments are more effective than others. Their simulations replicate the patterns of success and failure found in the developmental literature, and provide explicit computational insights into exactly why the interventions that include training on spelling-sound regularities are more effective than those focusing on phonological development alone.

In the study presented below, we hypothesize that specific audio-visual training designed to improve phonetic feature perception could help dyslexic children to specify phonemic representations. Consequently, they should not confuse close phonemes on the phonetic features which could facilitate written word processing. To our knowledge, no computer-based training using the simultaneous presentation of phonological units and orthographic units has been used with children with reading disabilities. We further hypothesized that audio-visual training will boost matching between visuo-orthographic patterns and phonological units. In other words, the phonological impairment concerning voicing which is characteristic of dyslexic children might be alleviated by means of audio-visual training which requires these children to process phonetic features both in the visual and auditory modalities.

In a first exploratory, controlled study (Magnan, Ecalle, Veuillet &and Collet, 2004), we trained 14 dyslexic children attending a specialized primary school with daily specific audio-visual training sessions designed to support phonetic feature perception. The results indicate the impact of audio-visual training on performances in a silent word reading task. The aim of this study was to evaluate the feasibility of this method in a more ordinary environment with older children. The training sessions therefore took place in a secondary school with older dyslexic children. Moreover, the effect of the training was studied in a reading aloud task and in a sentence comprehension task. Finally, a different design was used in the experiment presented here. In the previous study, all the dyslexics were trained using the audio-visual method, whereas a distinction is made between two different kinds of training here: one involving audio-visual voicing exercises and another taking the form of a multimedia "talking book" which provided a narrative context for the reading activity.

To promote motivation, audio-visual training was provided in relatively short chunks (15 minutes), and the task was integrated into a computer game with graphics designed by a commercial game developer (*Play-On*, :, Barbier & Danon-Boileau &and Barbier, 2000). Furthermore, in line with a recent study (Zellweger &and Mackinlay, 2000), we chose to use digitized speech to assist developing readers. These authors think that speech synthesis technology is not of high enough quality for use with dyslexic children. When the main purpose of the supporting speech support is to assist in decoding, i.e. the comprehension of the letter-sound correspondence, the low quality of speech synthesis could well constitute a problem.

TRAINING WITH DYSLEXIC CHILDREN: A NEW STUDY

Participants

Sixteen dyslexic children were selected from a dyslexic population at a secondary school. They had normal or corrected-to-normal vision and no neurological deficits or overt physical handicap. From this group, all the children who met the following two criteria were selected: an overall IQ score of 70 or more on the French version of the WISC-R and reading retardation of at least 24 months behind their chronological age (see Table 1). These children were separated into two equal groups with the same chronological age (13;4 years old.), i.e. an experimental group and a control group (Table 1). The two subgroups were strictly matched on educational and cognitive levels as well as for their reading level which was assessed just before the training using a standardized word reading test (Lefavrais, 1965). No significant difference ($p>.10$) was found on lexical age or on non-verbal intelligence scores assessed with the Progressive Matrices Standard PM 38 (Raven, Court, &and Raven, 1998).

A set of neuropsychological and phonological tests was administered to each individual by therapists before the experiment. These tests are routinely used to assess reading-impaired children in French dyslexic centers. Thus the children who participated in this study were carefully identified as exhibiting only a reading impairment.

In the secondary school in question, reading was taught with an emphasis on grapheme-to-phoneme conversion and reading out loud rather than whole-word recognition and silent reading for comprehension. Our sample of sixteen dyslexics had been selected by their education authority to receive similar remedial teaching. This remedial teaching represented an extension of the mixed approach to reading instruction.

A set of neuropsychological and phonological tests was administered to each individual by therapists before the experiment. These tests are routinely used to assess reading-impaired children in French dyslexic centers. Thus the children who participated in this study were carefully identified as exhibiting only a reading impairment.

In the secondary school in question, reading was taught with an emphasis on grapheme-to-phoneme conversion and reading out loud rather than whole-word recognition and silent reading for comprehension. Our sample of sixteen dyslexics had been selected by their education authority to receive similar remedial teaching. This remedial teaching represented an extension of the mixed approach to reading instruction.

Table 1. Descriptive data for subjects in the experimental and control groups at the onset of the study

	subjects	chronological age	lexical age	PM test
experimental group	S1	157	96	37
	S2	168	85	42
	S3	141	113	28
	S4	170	87	30
	S5	157	95	25
	S6	159	83	35
	S7	171	97	41
	S8	160	99	40
control group	S9	145	104	21
	S10	158	93	38
	S11	158	97	50
	S12	150	89	33
	S13	155	122	38
	S14	176	93	40
	S15	172	86	26
	S16	161	99	45

Notes: Lexical age was assessed with the "Alouette" reading test (Lefavrais, 1965); non verbal intelligence was assessed with Raven Progressive Matrices.

Procedure

A traditional pre-test, training phase, post-test design was used in this study. The sixteen children received half an hour of training every day (2 short sessions of 15 minutes each) over a period of five weeks. They thus received a total of 10 hours of training. Eight children (experimental group) received audio-visual training on the discrimination of the phonetic feature of voicing. The other eight (control group) used a computerized "talking book" program. All the children were trained individually using one exercise (discrimination or talking book) from the program developed by Danon-Boileau and Barbier (2000). During the training period, the children were not administered any other phonological training program.

The audio-visual training focused on paired-item voicing oppositions and involved six pairs of phonemes: /p/-/b/; /t/-/d/; /k/-/g/; /f/-/v/; /s/-/z/ et /ch/-/j/. The participants listened to a CV syllable (/pa/) and decided between two printed alternatives (*pa* or *ba*) which differed in their voicing. Immediately after the participants had listened to the syllable, a basket-ball fell from the top of screen and the child pressed one of two keys (left or right) to put the ball in the basket corresponding to *pa* or *ba* (see Figure 1).

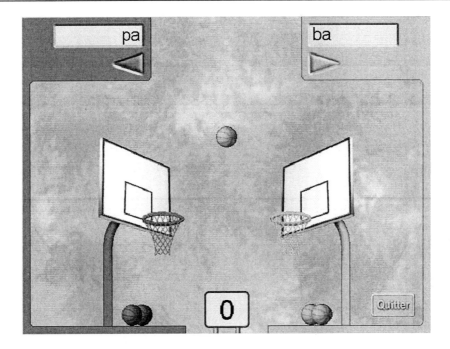

Figure 1. A computer screenshot of the animated multimedia syllable discrimination task

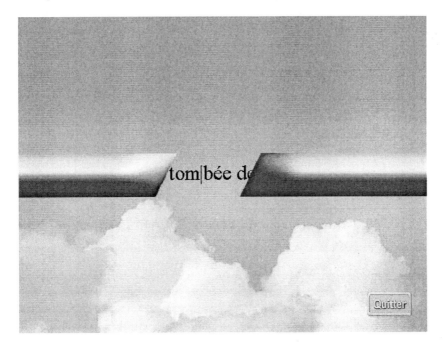

Figure 2. A computer screenshot of the animated multimedia talking book

The computerized "talking book" program enabled the children to read texts on the computer screen under whole word and syllable speech feedback conditions (see Figure 2). The reading material consisted of a set of short stories selected from children's literature.

Tests

The participants were tested individually over two sessions during normal school hours, the first session being administered before and the second one after training. Two reading tests were administered: a word reading test and a comprehension reading test.

Word Reading Test

This test was taken from the BELEC, a test battery designed to help in the assessment of the cognitive processes involved in the reading and spelling abilities of French-speaking children (Mousty &and Leybaert, 1999). These sub-tests were designed in such a way to make it possible to measure the effect of several psycholinguistic variables (such as word frequency, orthographic regularity, syllabic complexity, word length and lexicality). Only the reading subtests referred to as MIM and REGUL were used. MIM consists of reading aloud 72 items, 48 words and 24 pseudowords. Two series of items, A and B, composed of strictly matched items were proposed, series A during the pre-test session and series B during the post-test session. In the REGUL subtest, the children had to read aloud 24 words and 24 irregular words. For both subtests, only the global scores were taken into account in this study.

Comprehension Test

This test was adapted from the TROG (Test for Reception of Grammar; Bishop, 1983). The children had to read silently a sentence printed under four pictures and choose the picture that corresponded to the sentence. Twenty sentences had to be read. This test, called E20 (Khomsi, 1990), is used for children from 7 to 14 years old.

Results

The descriptive data are presented in Table 2. For each reading test, an ANOVA with a between-factor group (experimental *vs.* control) and a within-factor session (session 1 *vs* session 2) was carried out on the global scores. The interaction between the factors should provide evidence for an effect of training.

Table 2. Mean scores (standard deviations) in the reading tests (with maximum) for the experimental and control groups in the two sessions

	Word reading				Reading comprehension	
	MIM (/72)		REGUL (/48)		E20 (/20)	
	session 1	session 2	session 1	session 2	session 1	session 2
exp	46.3 (8.2)	54 (8.4)	36 (6.2)	40.1 (4.8)	16.1 (1.5)	16.4 (1.4)
cont	54 (4.7)	57.1 (2.1)	40.1 (4.5)	40.6 (3.6)	14.8 (1.8)	15.6 (1.5)

In the MIM subtest, the Group*Session interaction was significant, $F(1, 14) = 4.67, p =.$ 05, $\eta^2 = .25$. The interaction was due to the fact that the scores increasing more steeply in the experimental group (+ 7.7), t(7) = 5.64, $p = .0008, d = .87$, than in the control group (+3.1), t(7) = 1.15, ns. Moreover, in session 1, the control group significantly outperformed the experimental group, t(14) = 2.31, $p = .04, d = -1.02$, whereas in session 2 the difference between the scores was not significant ($p>.10$).

In the REGUL sub-test, the Group*Session interaction was significant, $F(1, 14) = 10.1, p =. 007, \eta^2 = .72$. The interaction was due to the fact that the scores increased more sharply in the experimental group (+ 4.1), t(7) = 1.81, $p =.11, d = .72$, than in the control group (+0.5), t(7) = 0.28, ns. At Nevertheless, no statistical difference was found ($p>.10$) between the groups at sessions 1 and 2. Finally, in the comprehension test, the ANOVA revealed no interaction between group and session factors.

CONCLUSION

This study has shown that training using a computer game incorporating an audio-visual phoneme discrimination task improved reading skills. The effectiveness of the present training program during the relatively short training period might be attributable to two factors. First, the training proposed in this study required the children to process phonetic features. In line with the phonetic model (Rosen, 2003),, we think that the phonological deficits in dyslexic children may be partly due to impairments in the phonetic organization of phoneme detectors (Serniclaes et al., 2001). Second, this type of training leads children to establish a link between print and phonology and helps them to develop ortho-phonological representations in accordance with a connectionist model of reading development and, more precisely, with the "mapping hypothesis" (Harm &and Seidenberg, 1999; 2004). Our training required the children to process this phonetic feature both in the visual and auditory modalities and we hypothesize that a this type of audio-visual training boosted the matching between visuo-orthographic patterns and phonological units.

Our empirical observations are consistent with two recent quantitative meta-analyses (Bus &and Ijzendoorn, 1999; Ehri et al., 2001) and with reading interventions simulated with an actual connectionist model of reading development (Harm et al., 2003). These simulations replicated the empirical findings, thus indicating that remediations that include training on spelling-sound regularities are more effective than those targeting phonological awareness alone.

Some researchers have argued that there are developmental, age-related boundaries beyond which the remediation of dyslexic children on the basis of phonological training is no longer possible (Wagner, Torgersen &and Rashotte, 1994). However, other authors (Lovett &and Steinbach, 1997; Tijms, Hoeks, Paulussen-Hoogeboom &and Smolenaars, 2003) have shown that the effectiveness of training does not decrease with increasing age. The current study extends these findings by showing that adolescents profit from training as much as elementary-school children do (Magnan et al., 2004; Magnan &and Ecalle, in press).

The literature on the use of phonological training to treat reading impairments is extensive. Numerous studies have evaluated the potential of so-called computer-based reading instruction. (e.g., Lewin, 2000; McKenna, Reinking &and Labbo, 1997; Wise et al.,

1999; 2000). This training uses different approaches, including the teacher and computer-delivered instruction of syllable manipulation and grapheme–phoneme matching. These studies have not focused on any specific deficit and have concentrated particularly on poor readers. Most of the studies have simply compared children who have been exposed to different forms of speech segmentation. Thus the study conducted by Wise *et al.* (1999) focused on three versions of phonological training. Few studies have used a strictly matched control group, or a group that has not been exposed to computer learning at all. In well-controlled studies, intensive phonological training has been found to increase phonological awareness and sometimes reading, although the mechanisms underpinning this improvement remain unclear.

Thus, most of the programs designed to investigate the question of literacy possess numerous components, including auditory processing training, phonological processing training, attention and memory training, and many other specific cognitive processes that are manipulated by the program (Cohen Plaza, Perez-Diaz, Lanthier, Chauvin, Hambourg, *et al.,* in press).

Our data come from a study of treatment designed to test the specific theoretical hypothesis that there is a speech-specific failure in phonological representations in developmental dyslexia. Consequently, our remediation has targeted one specific issue and has focused on the presumed underlying deficit. Like the study reported here, many researchers have taken a specific component as their starting point: visual strategy (Geiger, Lettvin, &and Fahle, 1994), phonemic awareness (Hecht &and Close, 2002), perceptual temporal processing of auditory stimuli (Merzenich *et al.*, 1996; Tallal *et al.,* 1996), perceptual processing with non-linguistic audio-visual stimuli (Kujala, Karma, Cepionene, Belitz, Turkkila, Tervaniemi, &and Näätänen, 2001), cognitive strategies (Das, Mishra, &and Pool, 1995), motor control (McPhillips, Hepper, &and Mulhem, 2000), phonological awareness and naming speed (Wolf, Miller, &and Donelly, 2000). In this study, we adopted a more focused perspective by investigating whether audio-visual training directed specifically at improving phonemic processing can enhance reading skills.

As far as we know, no computer-based training involving the simultaneous presentation of phonemic units and orthographic units has been used to study dyslexic children within the framework of this perspective. In a recent study, Moore, Rosenberg and Coleman (2005) have shown that auditory training with a computer game incorporating an adaptive phoneme discrimination task improved phonological awareness and word listening skills in 8 to 10-year-old mainstream school children. These authors dido not assessed the reading skills after training. Unfortunately, this auditory training has not been used with dyslexic children.

Our research has shown that, following intensive and short training, it is possible to improve reading skills. A short period of intensive training on a task involving the matching of visual and auditory sequential patterns was found to improve reading. One characteristic of the program used here is the brief period of training. Some studies also suggest that long and elaborate training may not be necessary to bring about improvements in reading skills (Kujala *et al.,* 2001 ; Agnew, Dorn &and Eden, 2004). From an applied perspective, this aspect of the training is very important.

One question is left unanswered by this study and we plan to address this in future research. We do not know whether this audio-visual training induces a temporary benefit or a permanent improvement. Most studies have evaluated the short-term effectiveness of training (Lyon &and Moats, 1997). A small number of long-term studies have recently been conducted (Elbro &and Petersen, 2004; Tijms, Hoeks, Paulussen-Hoogeboom, &and Smolenaars, 2003; Torgersen, Alexander, Wagner, Rashotte, Voeller, &and Conway, 2001; Wise *et al.,* 1999). It is clear that the aim of any treatment that is administered is to bring about a lasting improvement. In order to shed light on this question, we plan to re-assess subjects' reading skills some months after the end of the remediation program. Moreover, word identification is evidently not sufficient for reading. Reading also involves the use of syntactic rules and the assimilation of the specific characteristics of written texts. In line with the phonological model of dyslexia, we think that dyslexic children experience difficulties with written language because their ability to segment written words into phonemes is impaired, thus preventing word identification. This low-level phonological deficit prevents words from reaching the high-level linguistic processing which would allow the reader to obtain meaning from the text. Thus, most dyslexics have intact memory and language comprehension processes which remain unactivated because they can only be activated after a word has been identified through phonological processing. To assess the effectiveness of a treatment properly, it is not sufficient simply to observe significant improvements in word recognition. It is also necessary to establish that a functional level of reading has been achieved. Thus, future research must address the long-term effects of training on reading comprehension tasks.

However, the present results are encouraging with respect to both the understanding and remediation of dyslexia. The possibility that computer-based learning as described here could be used either as part of or in addition to the school curriculum has implications for educational resourcing and teaching methods. Computer-assisted instruction can be used to improve the learning experience and the performance of children with reading and writing difficulties. Nowadays, computers are an integral part of the daily life of many children, and we must ensure that the use of computer-assisted learning in the classroom will prove to be an asset for poor readers and writers. We know that children with reading and writing difficulties are motivated by certain uses of computer technology, and this fact must be exploited to ensure the greatest benefit to struggling readers. Moreover, in clinical practice, reading therapy is individualized, and adapted to the patient depending on his/her deficit. This type of audio-visual training method could be used by speech-therapist for developing reading skills in children undergoing speech and language therapy.

ACKNOWLEDGEMENTS

We are very grateful to Damien Houdou and the staff of the "Sainte Thérèse" secondary school on Laval, France, and to Marlène Mahot, a student who participated in this study.

REFERENCES

Adlard, A., &and Hazan, V. (1998). Speech perception abilities in children with specific reading difficulties (dyslexia). *Quarterly Journal of Experimental Psychology, 51A*, 153–177.

Ahissar, M., Protopapas, A., Reid, M., &and Merzenich, M.M. (2000). Auditory processing parallels reading abilities in adults. *Proceedings of the National Academy of Sciences of the United States of America, 97,* 6832–6837.

Beck, I. (1989). *Reading Today and Tomorrow (Teachers' Editions for Grades 1 and 2).* Austin, Texas: Holt and Co.

Beck, I., &and Hamilton, R. (2000). *Beginning reading module.* Washington D.C: American Federation of Teachers.

Bishop, D.V.M. (1983). *TROG. Test for Reception of Grammar.* Medical Research Council. University of Manchester. Chapel Press.

Blomert, L., &and Mitterer, H. (2004). The fragile nature of the speech-perception deficit in dyslexia: Natural vs. synthetic speech. *Brain Language, 89,* 21-26.

Bradley, L., &and Bryant, P.E. (1983). Categorizing sounds and learning to read: A causal connection. *Nature, 301,* 419-421.

Bryant, P. E., &and Bradley, L. (1985). *Children's reading problems.* Oxford: Basil Blackwell.

Bus, A.G., &and van Ijzendoorn, M.H. (1999). Phonological awareness and early reading: A meta-analysis of experimental training studies. *Journal of Educational Psychology, 91,* 403-414.

Castles, A., &and Coltheart, M. (2004). Is there a causal link from phonological awareness to success in learning to read ? *Cognition, 91,* 77-111.

Chera, P., &and Wood, C. (2003). Animated multimedia "talking books" can promote phonological awareness in children beginning to read. *Learning and Instruction, 13,* 33-52.

Cohen, D., Plaza, M., Perez-Diaz, F., Lanthier, O., Chauvin, D., Hambourg, N., Wilson, A.J., Basquin, M., Mazet, P., &and Rivière, J.P. (in press). Individual cognitive training of reading disability improves word identification and sentence comprehension in adults with mild mental retardation. *Research in Developmental Disabilities.*

Danon-Boileau, L., &and Barbier, D. (2000). *Play-On: Un logiciel d'entraînement à la lecture.* [A training program for children with difficulties in learning to read]. Paris: AudiviMédia.

Das, J.P., Mishra, R.K., &and Pool, J.E. (1995). An experiment on cognitive remediation of word-reading difficulty. *Journal of Learning Disability, 8,* 66–79

Ehri, L.C., Nunes, S.R., Stahl, S., &and Willows, D.M. (2001). Systematic phonics instruction helps students learn to read: Evidence from the National Reading Panel's meta-analysis. *Review of Educational Research, 71,* 393-447.

Elbro, C. &and Petersen, D.K. (2004). Long-term effects of phoneme awareness and letter sound training: An intervention study with children at risk for dyslexia. *Journal of Educational Psychology, 96 (4),* 660-670.

Agnew, J.A., Dorn, C., &and Eden, G.F. (2004). Effect of intensive training on auditory processing and reading skills, *Brain and Language, 88,* 21-25.

Elbro, C., Rasmussen, I., &and Spelling, B. (1996). Teaching reading to disabled readers with language disorders: A controlled evaluation of synthetic speech feedback. *Scandinavian Journal of Psychology, 37,* 140-155

Farmer, M.E., &and Klein, R.M. (1995). The evidence for a temporal processing deficit linked to dyslexia: A review. *Psychonomic Bulletin &and Review, 2(4),* 460-493.

Fawcett, A. (Ed.) (2001). *Dyslexia, theory and good practice.* London: Whurr.

Frith, U. (1997). Brain, mind and behaviour in dyslexia. In C. Hulme &and M.J. Snowling (Eds.), *Dyslexia: Biology, cognition and intervention* (pp. 1-19). London: Whurr.

Geiger, G., Lettvin, J.Y., &and Fahle, M. (1994). Dyslexic children learn a new visual strategy for reading: A controlled experiment. *Vision Research, 34,* 1223-1233

Goswami, U. (2000). The potential of a neuro-constructivist framework for developmental dyslexia: The abnormal development of phonological representations? *Developmental Science, 3,* 27-29.

Goswami, U., &and Bryant, P.E. (1990). *Phonological skills and learning to read.* Hillsdale, NJ: Erlbaum.

Harm, M., &and Seidenberg, M.S. (1999). Phonology, reading acquisition, and dyslexia: Insights from connectionist models. *Psychological Review, 106,* 491-528.

Harm, M., &and Seidenberg, M.S. (2004). Computing the meanings of words in reading: Cooperative division of labor between visual and phonological processes. *Psychological Review, 111,* 662-720.

Harm, M., McCandliss, B., &and Seidenberg, M. (2003). Modelling the successes and failures of interventions for disabled readers. *Scientific Studies of Reading, 7,* 155-182.

Hecht, S.A. &and Close, L. (2002) Emergent literacy skills and training time uniquely predict variability in responses to phonemeic awareness training in disadvantaged kindergartners. *Journal of Experimental Child Psychology, 82,* 93-115.

Hulme, C., &and Snowling, M. (Eds.) (1997). *Dyslexia: Biology, cognition and intervention.* London: Whurr.

Jorm, A.F., Share, D.L., MacLean, R., &and Matthews, R.G. (1984). Phonological recoding skills and learning to read: A longitudinal study. *Applied Psycholinguistics, 5,* 201-207.

Khomsi, A. (1990). *Epreuve d'évaluation de la compétence en lecture: E 20.*[Comprehension reading test]. Paris: ECPA.

Kujala, T., Karma, K., Cepionene, R., Belitz, S., Turkkila, P., Tervaniemi, M., &and Näätänen, R. (2001). Plastic neural changes and reading improvement caused by audiovisual training in reading-impaired children. *Proceedings of the National Academy of Sciences, 98(18),* 10509-10514.

Lefavrais, P. (1965). *Le test de l'Alouette* [Reading test]. Paris: ECPA.

Lewin, C. (2000). Exploring the effects of talking book software in UK primary classrooms. *Journal of Research in Reading, 23(2),* 149-157.

Lovett, M.W., &and Steinbach, K.A. (1997). The effectiveness of remedial programs for reading disabled children of different ages : Does the benefit decrease for older children? *Learning Disability Quarterly, 20,* 189-210.

Lyon, G.R, &and Moats, L.C. (1997). Critical conceptual and methodological considerations in reading interventions research. *Journal of Learning Disabilities, 30, 578-588.*

Magnan, A., &and Ecalle, J. (in press). Audio-visual training in children with reading disabilities. *Computers &and Education.*

Magnan, A., &and Ecalle, J., Veuillet, E., &and Collet, L. (2004). The effects of an audio-visual training program in dyslexic children. *Dyslexia, 10,* 131-140.

Manis, F.R., Seidenberg, M.S., Doi, L. M., McBride-Chang, C, &and Petersen, A. (1996). On the bases of two subtypes of developmental dyslexia. *Cognition, 58,* 157-195.

Mann, V. (1984). Longitudinal prediction and prevention of early reading difficulty. *Annals of Dyslexia, 34,* 117–136.

Marshall, C.M., Snowling, M.J., &and Bailey, P.J. (2001). Rapid auditory processing and phonological ability in normal readers and readers with dyslexia. *Journal of Speech Language and Hearing Research, 44*, 925–940.

McAnally, K. I., &and Stein, J. F. (1996). Auditory temporal coding in dyslexia. *Proceedings of the Royal Society of London Series B-Biological Sciences, 263*, 961–965.

McCandliss, B.D., Beck, I., Sandak, R., &and Perfetti, C. (2003). Focusing attention on decoding for children with poor reading skills: A study of the Word Building Intervention. *Scientific Studies of Reading, 3*, 75-104.

McKenna M.C., D. Reinking, L.D., &and Labbo, (1997). Using talking books with reading-disabled students. *Reading and Writing Quarterly. 13(2)*, 185-190.

McPhillips, M., Hepper, P.G., &and Mulhem, G. (2000). Effects of replicating primary-reflex movements on specific reading difficulties in children: A randomised, double-blind, control trial. *Lancet, 355*, 537–541.

Merzenich, M.M., Jenkins, W.M., Johnston, P., Schreiner, C., Miller, S.L., &and Tallal, P. (1996). Temporal processing deficits of language-learning impaired children ameliorated by training. *Science, 271*, 77-81.

Mioduser, D., Tur-Kaspa, H., &and Leitner, I. (2000). The learning value of computer-based instruction of early reading skills. *Journal of Computer Assisted Learning, 16*, 54-63.

Mitchell, M.J., &and Fox, B.J. (2001). The effects of computer software for developing awareness in low-progress readers. *Reading Research and Instruction, 40*, 315-331.

Mody, M., Studdert-Kennedy, M., &and Brady, S. (1997). Speech perception deficits in poor readers: Auditory processing or phonological coding ? *Journal of Experimental Child Psychology, 64*, 199-231.

Moore, D.R., Rosenberg, J.F., &and Coleman, J.S. (2005). Discrimination training of phonemic contrasts enhances phonological processing in mainstream school children. *Brain and Language, 94*, 72-85.

Morais, J. (2003). Levels of phonological representation in skilled reading and in learning to read. *Reading and Writing, 16*, 123-151.

Mousty, P., &and Leybaert, J. (1999). Evaluation des habiletés de lecture et d'orthographe au moyen de la BELEC: données longitudinales auprès d'enfants francophones testés en 2ème et 4ème années. [Evaluation of reading and spelling ability by means of the BELEC]. *Revue Européenne de Psychologie Appliquée, 49(4)*, 325-342.

Nagarajan, S., Mahncke, H., Salz, T., Tallal, P., Roberts, T., &and Merzenich, M.M. (1999) *Proceedings of National Academy of Science, 96*, 6483-6488

Nittrouer, S. (1999). Do temporal processing deficits cause phonological processing problems? *Journal of Speech, Language, and Hearing Research, 42*, 925-942.

Olofsson, A. (1992). Synthetic speech and computer aided reading for reading disabled children. *Reading and Writing, 4*, 165-178.

Olson, R.K., &and Wise, B.W. (1992). Reading on the computer with orthographic and speech feedback: An overview of the Colorado Remedial Reading Project. *Reading and Writing, 4*, 107-144.

Olson, R.K., Foltz, G., &and Wise, B. (1986). Reading instruction and remediation with the aid of computer speech. *Behavior Research Methods, Instruments, and Computers, 18*, 93-99.

Olson, R.K., Wise, B.W., Ring, J., &and Johnson, M. (1997). Computer-based remedial training in phoneme awareness and phonological decoding: Effects on the post-training development on word recognition. *Scientific Studies of Reading, 1*, 235-253.

Ramus, F. (2001). Dyslexia-talk of two theories. *Nature, 412*, 393–395.

Ramus, F. (2003). Developmental dyslexia: Specific phonological deficit or general sensorimotor dysfunction? *Current Opinion in Neurobiology, 13*, 212–218..

Ramus, F., Rosen, S., Dakin, S.C., Day, B.L., Castellote, J.M., White, S., &and Frith, U. (2003). Theories of developmental dyslexia: Insights from a multiple case study of dyslexic adults. *Brain, 126*, 841–865.

Raven, J.C., Court, J.H., &and Raven, J. (1998). *Progressive Matrices Standard, Edition 1998*. Paris: EAP.

Rayner, K., Foorman, B.R., Perfetti, C.A., Pesetsky, D., &and Scidenberg, M.S. (2001). How psychological science informs the teaching of reading. *Psychological Science in the Public Interest, 2*, 31-74.

Rosen, S. (2003). Auditory processing in dyslexia and specific language impairment: Is there a deficit ? What is its nature ? Does it explain anything ? *Journal of Phonetics, 31*, 509-527.

Rosen, S., &and Manganari, E. (2001). Is there a relationship between speech and nonspeech auditory processing in children with dyslexia ? *Journal of Speech Language and Hearing Research, 44(4)*, 720-736.

Seidenberg, M.S., &and MacClelland, J.L. (1989). A distributed, developmental model of word recognition and naming. *Psychological Review, 96*, 523-568.

Serniclaes, W., Sprenger-Charolles, L., Carré, R., &and Démonet, J.-F. (2001). Perceptual discrimination of speech sounds in developmental dyslexia. *Journal of Speech, Language and Hearing Research, 44*, 384-399.

Serniclaes, W., Van Heghe, S., Mousty, P., Carré, R., &and Sprenger-Charolles, L. (2004). Allophonic mode of speech perception in dyslexia. *Journal of Experimental Child Psychology, 87*, 336-361.

Shankweiler, D., &and Liberman, I.Y. (1989). *Phonology and reading disability*. Ann Arbor, MI: University Michigan Press.

Share, D.L., Jorm, A.F., MacLean, R., &and Matthews, R. (2002). Temporal processing and reading disability. *Reading and Writing: An Interdisciplinary Journal, 15*, 151–178.

Share, D.L. (1995). Phonological recoding and self-teaching: Sine qua non of reading acquisition. *Cognition, 55*, 151-218.

Shaywitz, S.E. (1998) Dyslexia. *New England Journal of Medicine,. 338*, 307-312.

Snowling, M.J. (1998). Dyslexia as a phonological deficit: Evidence and implications. *Child Psychology &and Psychiatry Review, 3*, 4-11.

Snowling, M.J. (2000). *Dyslexia*. Oxford: Blackwell.

Stanovich, K., Siegel, L.S. &and Gottardo, A. (1997). Progress in the search for dyslexia subtypes. In C. Hulme &and M.J. Snowling (Eds.), *Dyslexia: Biology, cognition and intervention* (pp. 108-130). London: Whurr.

Stanovich, K.E., &and Siegel, L.S. (1994). Phenotypic performance profile of children with reading disabilities: A regression based test of the phonological-core variable difference model. *Journal of Educational Psychology, 86*, 24-53.

Stein, J. (2001). The magnocellular theory of developmental dyslexia. *Dyslexia, 7*, 12-36.

Studdert-Kennedy, M., &and Mody, M. (1995). Auditory temporal perception deficits in the reading impaired: A critical review of the evidence. *Psychonomic Bulletin &and Review, 2,* 508-514.

Swan, D., &and Goswami, U. (1997). Phonological awareness deficits in developmental dyslexia and the phonological representations hypothesis. *Journal of Experimental Child Psychology, 66,* 18-41.

Tallal, P. (1980). Auditory temporal perception, phonics, and reading disabilities in children. *Brain and Language, 9,* 182-198.

Tallal, P., Miller, S., Bedi, G., Byma, G., Wang, X., Nagarajan, S., Schreiner, C., Jenkins, W.M. &and Mezernich, M.M. (1996). Language comprehension in language-learning impaired children improved with acoustically modified speech. *Science, 271,* 81-84.

Temple, E. (2002). Brain mechanisms in normal and dyslexic readers. *Current Opinion in Neurobiology,. 12,* 178-83.

Tijms, J., Hoeks, J.J., Paulussen-Hoogeboom, M.C., &and Smolenaars, A.J. (2003). Long-term effects of a psycholinguistic treatment for dyslexia. *Journal of Research in Reading, 26(2),* 121-140.

Torgersen, J.K., Alexander, A.W., Wagner, R.K., Rashotte, C.A., Voeller, K.K.S, &and Conway, T. (2001). Intensive remedial instruction for children with severe reading disabilities: Immediate and long-term outcomes from two instructional approaches. *Journal of Learning Disabilities, 34,* 33-58.

Torgesen, J. K. (1999). Phonologically based reading disabilities: Toward a coherent theory of one kind of learning disability. In R.J. Sternberg &and L. Spear-Swerling (Eds.), *Perspectives on learning disabilities* (pp. 231-262). New Haven: Westview Press.

Torgesen, J.K., &and Barker, T. (1995). Computers as aids in the prevention and remediation of reading disabilies. *Learning Disabilities Quarterly, 18,* 76-88.

Van Daal, V.H.P., &and Reitsma, P. (1990). Effects of independent word practice with segmented and whole word sound feedback in disabled readers. *Journal of Research in Reading, 13,* 133-148.

Van Daal, V.H.P., Reitsma, P., &and Van Der Leig, A. (1994). Processing units in word reading by disabled readers. *Journal of Experimental Child Psychology (57),* 180-210.

Wagner, R.K., Torgersen, J.K., &and Rashotte, C.A. (1994). Development of reading-related phonological processing abilities: New evidence of bi-directional causality from a latent variable longitudinal study. *Developmental Psychology, 30,* 73-87.

Wise, B.W., Olson, R. (1995). Computer-based phonological awareness and reading instruction. *Annals of Dyslexia, 45,* 99-122.

Wise, B.W., Ring, J., &and Olson, R.K. (1999). Training phonological awareness with and without attention to articulation. *Journal of Experimental Child Psychology, 72,* 271-304.

Wise, B.W., Ring, J., &and Olson, R.K. (2000). Individual differences in gains from computer-assisted remedial reading with more emphasis on phonological analysis or accurate reading in context. *Journal of Experimental Child Psychology, 77,* 197-235.

Wolf, M., Miller, L., &and Donelly, K. (2000). Retrieval, Automaticity, Vocabulary Elaboration, Orthography (RAVE-O): A comprehensive, fluency-based reading intervention program. *Journal of Learning Disabilities, 33,* 375–386.

Zellweger, P., &and MacKinlay, J.D. (2000). The fluid reading primer: Animated decoding support for emergent readers. *Proceedings of ED-MEDIA 2001,* Tampere, Finland.

In: Dyslexia in Children: New Research
Editor: Christopher B. Hayes, pp. 65-78

ISBN 1-59454-969-9
© 2006 Nova Science Publishers, Inc.

Chapter 3

CROSS-MODAL TEMPORAL DYSFUNCTION IN CHILDREN WITH DYSLEXIA: IS AGE A MEDIATING FACTOR?

Sabine Heim, Andreas Keil and Martina Ruf

Department of Psychology, University of Konstanz, Konstanz, Germany

ABSTRACT

Developmental dyslexia has been associated with an auditory rate processing deficit as part of a cross-modal temporal dysfunction. The empirical evidence for the co-occurrence of visual and auditory impairments is not conclusive, however. One possibility is that the discordant findings are moderated by the subject's age. Here, we investigate cross-sectionally whether a visual temporal deficit in children with dyslexia disappears through development. The same experimental tasks as used in an earlier study involving 13-year-olds were administered to 11 year-old dyslexic and normally literate children. Auditory rate processing was assessed by means of a syllable-discrimination task; visual processing was indexed by judgments of temporal order of lightness changes. As a main result, dyslexic children exhibited higher visual thresholds than the controls did. This was in contrast to what was observed in older participants. Auditory data of young and older dyslexic children yielded two subgroups: one benefiting from temporal extension of stop consonant-vowel syllables and the other showing a balanced performance profile across consonant durations. Both younger dyslexics and older controls demonstrated no relationship between auditory accuracy and visual thresholds. In contrast, significant relationships were found in the younger control and older dyslexic group. The findings suggest the co-occurrence of visual and auditory impairments in young children with dyslexia. Visual processing deficits, however, seem to ameliorate across development. Hence, younger dyslexic children may have deficits in both modalities, but older dyslexics may not show co-occurrence of visual and auditory impairments.

INTRODUCTION

Developmental dyslexia is a language-based learning disorder that affects an individual's written language skills, despite adequate intellectual capacity, education, and sociocultural opportunity (Dilling, Mombour, and Schmidt, 1991). The core problem in dyslexia has been considered linguistic in origin and manifests itself as a disability in representation and processing of speech sounds (Goswami, 2000; Snowling, 2000). Tallal (1980) has proposed that these phonological difficulties result from an impairment to process brief or rapid successive auditory cues. Originally, Tallal's research focused on children with specific language impairment (SLI), a condition characterized by significant deficits in oral language ability in the absence of extraneous factors. In a seminal set of studies, Tallal and Piercy (1973a,b; 1974; 1975) found the difficulties of SLI children to arise in tasks that required discriminating and sequencing rapidly occurring tones or tones having a short duration. This deficit was in the range of some tens of milliseconds, leading them to focus on the phoneme level of speech. In particular, stop consonants such as /b/ and /d/ are characterized by brief transitional periods during which the frequencies of the formants change very rapidly over time. Accordingly, SLI children had problems differentiating stop consonant-vowel syllables /ba/ and /da/, having consonant durations of 43 ms. They succeeded, however, when this time period was artificially extended to 95 ms.

More than 50% of children having SLI continue on to develop dyslexia (Stark et al., 1984; Tomblin, Zhang, Buckwalter, and Catts, 2000). Conversely, many dyslexic individuals, but by no means all, show deficits in parameters of oral language (Byrne, 1981; Joanisse, Manis, Keating, and Seidenberg, 2000). This relationship led Paula Tallal to assume that the auditory deficit may be causally related to both disorders. In fact, adaptive training of auditory rate processing has been shown to improve language and reading skills in children with SLI and dyslexia (Merzenich et al., 1996; Tallal et al., 1996; Temple et al., 2003). Children participated in training regimens, which used modified speech and non-speech stimuli. Initially, rapid transitional parts of the stimuli were prolonged in time and/or increased in amplitude. In addition, the temporal proximity between successive events was reduced. With children progressing and succeeding with tasks administered, the modified acoustic stimuli were presented at rates increasingly resembling those that occur in natural speech.

Poor temporal sensitivity in the visual modality has also been related to phonological difficulties present in dyslexic individuals. Specifically, accuracy in detecting visual coherent motion was correlated with performance in pseudoword reading, in both dyslexic and normal readers (Witton et al., 1998). This type of task involves detection of a subset of coherently moving elements in a pattern of randomly moving dots. Manipulating the percentage of coherently moving elements within a given frame, it is possible to determine thresholds for visual motion perception. Importantly, this procedure is highly sensitive to fast processes mediated by the visual magnocellular pathway of the central nervous system (Newsome and Paré, 1988; Shapley, 1990). Other measures, however, may reflect different aspects of processing speed and accuracy at high rates in the visual system. For instance, gap detection procedures and temporal-order judgments have been used in the visual domain (Farmer and Klein, 1993; 1995).

The issue of whether sensory problems are responsible for a phonological deficit is not decisive, however (Fitch and Tallal, 2003; Ramus, 2003). Moreover, there is a controversy concerning the putative co-occurrence of auditory and visual impairments in dyslexia. For instance, Van Ingelghem et al. (2001) found that 7 out of 10 dyslexic children had higher thresholds than normal readers both for auditory and visual gap detection. These authors employed white noise containing a silent interval (targets) amidst uninterrupted noise stimuli (standards) and double light flashes separated by a dark gap amidst single red lights, respectively. Participants were asked to identify the target stimuli in a forced choice design. Using different task paradigms, Heim, Freeman, Eulitz, and Elbert (2001) reported high-level visual performance in a small group of dyslexic children showing impaired discrimination of rapidly changing stop consonant-vowel syllables. The conflicting results could be related to characteristics of the sample, such as age, or the task difficulty, among others. From an early age, tasks of rate processing are subject to a pronounced developmental trajectory, being associated with the increasing ability to detect fast changes in the auditory environment (Benasich and Leevers, 2003). Accordingly, adults with a history of reading impairment may not show deficits in relatively simple tasks such as gap detection (McAnally and Stein, 1996; Protopapas, Ahissar, and Merzenich, 1997). The same may be true for older children with SLI (Bishop, Carlyon, Deeks, and Bishop, 1999). By contrast, more demanding acoustic tasks involving rapid, sequential, and brief stimuli continue to elicit higher thresholds in dyslexic adults (e.g., Hari and Kiesilä, 1996). Paralleling these observations, deficits in adults with dyslexia or poor decoding skills have been found more consistently in difficult visual tasks that require motion detection or identification (Conlon, Sanders, and Zapart, 2004; Talcott, Hansen, Assoku, and Stein, 2000; Wilmer, Richardson, Chen, and Stein, 2004; Witton et al., 1998). Di Lollo, Hanson, and McIntyre (1983) observed progressive improvement in visual gap detection from 8 to 14 years of age in dyslexic boys. No such trend was documented for normal readers. In a group suffering from SLI (Tallal, Stark, Kallman, and Mellits, 1981), 5- and 6-year-olds were found to be similarly impaired when responding to rapid successive stimuli presented to the auditory and visual modality. On the other hand, older affected individuals (7 and 8 years) made nearly twice as many errors in the auditory rather than visual task. Thus, it is conceivable that a visual deficit ameliorates or even disappears through development in certain individuals with language-based learning impairments.

In order to test the age hypothesis, the same auditory and visual tasks as used in an earlier study with on average 13.4-year-olds (Heim et al., 2001) were administered to a younger sample of children aged 11.5 years (significant age difference; $t(62) = 5.91$, $p < 0.001$). The tasks were selected to be representative for past work in the field. Although capturing meaningful variance of temporal auditory and visual processing (Fitch and Tallal, 2003), there are other possible tasks and indeed the choice of experimental design has been identified as crucial for investigations along the developmental trajectory of dyslexic individuals (Heim and Keil, 2004).

METHODS

Participants

Sixteen children (mean age 11.3 ± 1.1 years; 4 females) diagnosed with developmental dyslexia and 15 healthy control subjects (mean age 11.6 ± 1.1 years; 8 females) participated in the present study. All participants were native speakers of German and were reported having normal hearing and vision. Groups did not differ in terms of age and nonverbal intelligence as measured by Raven's Standard Progressive Matrices (Heller, Kratzmeier, and Lengfelder, 1998). Literacy skills were assessed by means of standardized tests of reading (Grissemann, 1998) and spelling (Grund, Haug, and Naumann, 1994; 1995; Müller, 1997; Rathenow, Laupenmühlen, and Vöge, 1981) as well as non-standardized word and pseudoword reading. Consistent with their difficulties, dyslexic children were significantly outperformed by the controls on all language tests (see Table 1).

Table 1. Psychometric data for the control and dyslexic groups (mean ± standard deviation, SD)

	Controls (n=15)	Dyslexics (n=16)	t-test	p
Non-verbal IQ	105.23 ± 13.57	97.97 ± 12.59	1.54	< 0.134
Standard word reading				
Errors	1.40 ± 1.64	7.81 ± 5.68	-4.33	< 0.001[#]
Time (s)	65.80 ± 25.87	122.88 ± 43.17	-4.50	< 0.001[#]
Standard passage reading				
Errors	8.53 ± 3.09	29.00 ± 15.17	-5.28	< 0.001[#]
Time (s)	139.07 ± 42.74	296.94 ± 110.64	-5.30	< 0.001[#]
Word reading				
Points (max.=150)	141.40 ± 6.71	125.31 ± 15.04	3.89	< 0.001[#]
Time (s)	59.27 ± 17.83	109.88 ± 43.21	-4.31	< 0.001[#]
Pseudoword reading				
Points (max.=150)	128.07 ± 11.07	95.38 ± 27.61	4.38	< 0.001[#]
Time (s)	106.87 ± 26.18	160.06 ± 59.81	-3.24	< 0.01[#]
Standard spelling				
Errors (ratio)	0.17 ± 0.13	0.58 ± 0.17	-7.47	< 0.001

[#] t-test is based on separate variance estimates

The study was approved by the ethics review board of the University of Konstanz. Written informed consent was obtained from the parents of the children prior to the experimental session. Children received shopping vouchers or cinema tickets for participating in the study.

Experimental Tasks

Two computer-based experimental tasks were implemented. The first (auditory) task required the child to press the right (green) response key if two successive syllables (/ba/-/ba/,

/da/-/da/) were the same and the left (red) key if they were different (/ba/-/da/, /da/-ba/). Syllables were created with a sampling rate of 10 kHz in a cascade mode by using SpeechLab software based on a Klatt formant synthesizer (Diesch, 1997). The total stimulus duration was 250 ms including a formant transition (FT) period of either 40 ms (rapid FT condition) or 90 ms (extended FT condition). Syllables shared identical fundamental frequency as well as the first, fourth, and fifth formants. Fundamental frequency started with a 5-ms delay at 128 Hz and decreased linearly to 109 Hz at syllable offset. The first formant had a starting frequency of 200 Hz sweeping up to a stationary frequency of 770 Hz within the FT periods. Onset frequencies of the second FT were 1095 Hz for /ba/ and 1702 Hz for /da/ reaching a stationary frequency of 1340 Hz. Corresponding transitional values for the third formant were 2100 and 2633 Hz, respectively, gliding to stationary 2400 Hz. The fourth and fifth formants were stationary at 3900 and 4600 Hz from stimulus onset.

The experimental procedure was identical for the rapid and extended FT conditions. The syllables were delivered to both ears via headphones with an intensity of 75 dB. Feedback was provided after each stimulus pair (= trial) by a happy or unhappy schematic face on the computer screen.

The training phase consisted of a maximum of 48 trials and finished if a criterion of 20 correct responses in 24 consecutive trials was achieved. During training an interstimulus interval (ISI) of 428 ms was employed; in the immediately following testing phase syllables were presented at six different ISIs: 8, 15, 30, 60, 150, and 305 ms (Tallal and Piercy, 1974, 1975). Testing included 48 trials with a randomized presentation of the different intervals. The percentages of correct trials were measured at each ISI.

In the second (visual) task, equiluminant light flashes of green and red were generated by two light-emitting diodes (LEDs). LEDs were mounted side by side (distance 1 cm) on a black surface slanted toward the subject. Subjects were asked to press either the red (left) or green (right) response key indicating the LED which flashed first. After the second LED flashed, both LEDs remained on for 2 s. Two-element stimulus sequences (red-green, green-red) were randomized across trials. During an initial training phase of 10 trials, onsets between two light flashes (SOA, stimulus onset asynchrony) varied between 310 and 400 ms, i.e., at rather long intervals, to allow all participants to understand the task. In the testing phase, the SOA was adjusted from trial to trial (starting SOA = 300 ms), using a staircase procedure. After one correct response in a given staircase, the SOA was shortened, whereas an incorrect answer led to the SOA being lengthened. Sizes of downward or upward steps were 10% of the previous value; below a 10-ms SOA a step size of 1 ms was used. The visual temporal-order threshold in milliseconds was defined as the arithmetic mean of the last 20 trials in the experiment, which began after completion of 10 downward and 10 upward steps.

RESULTS

In this section, we relate the results of two separate, cross-sectional studies using the same experimental procedures. First, indices of temporal dynamics in the visual system are reported, followed by auditory rate data. Effects of age and sensory modality are evaluated by relating the two samples and tasks, considering performance of dyslexic children, who did versus did not benefit from prolonged auditory stimulus durations.

Visual Performance

Capitalizing on a possible outgrow of a temporal deficit in the visual domain (see Introduction), we used a one-sided statistical approach to directly test the hypothesis that young dyslexic children may manifest elevated visual thresholds as compared to age controls. Unpaired t-test analysis showed a significant group difference in visual temporal-order thresholds (t(29) = -1.93; one-sided p < 0.05), indicating that dyslexic children (mean = 10.57, SD = 3.77) performed less well than control participants (mean = 8.02, SD = 3.59).

Auditory Performance

Auditory data were compared in mixed-design analysis of variance (ANOVA) with group (control, dyslexic) treated as between-subjects factor and FT condition (rapid, extended) and ISI (8, 15, 30, 60, 150, 305 ms) as within-subjects factors. Replicating previous results (Heim et al., 2001), dyslexics achieved lower accuracy scores than the controls did (group main effect, F(1,29) = 5.06; p < 0.05). Neither effects of FT condition and ISI nor any interaction fell within the range of statistical significance. However, there was a small tendency for larger group differences in the rapid than in the temporally extended FT condition (see Figure 1).

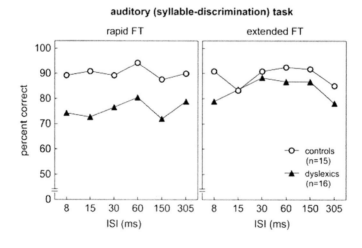

Figure 1. Percent correct responses for the control (open circles) and dyslexic (filled triangles) groups on the auditory syllable-discrimination task at various ISIs of the rapid and extended FT conditions.

Subgroup Analysis

Given the bimodal distribution of discrimination accuracy in the rapid FT condition, dyslexic subjects were classified into two groups using the same criteria as in the Heim et al. (2001) study. Since chance level was at 50%, we divided the above-chance range into 4 quartiles, of which the top quartile was considered to reflect good performance. Hence, dyslexic children scoring ≥ 87.5% at least in two of the shortest ISIs (8, 15, and 30 ms) were designated 'good perceivers', otherwise they were classified as 'poor perceivers'. Mixed-design ANOVA carried out with the three groups (controls, good/poor perceivers) yielded a significant group × FT condition interaction effect (F(2,28) = 9.16; p < 0.001). Furthermore, poor perceivers were significantly outperformed by the other groups (F(2,28) = 14.22; p < 0.001).

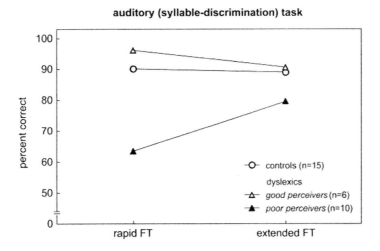

Figure 2. Percent correct responses in the auditory syllable-discrimination task for the control group (open circles) and dyslexic participants who were classified as good (open triangles) and poor (filled triangles) perceivers based on their performance in the three shortest ISIs of the rapid FT condition.

As depicted in Figure 2, the 6 dyslexic children (2 females) constituting the group of good perceivers did not differ from the controls in any of the conditions. However, the poor perceivers (n=10; 2 females) were significantly less accurate in the rapid FT condition compared to the other groups (Scheffé's ps < 0.01) and their performance level in the extended FT condition (Scheffé's p < 0.01).

Relationship between Visual and Auditory Rate Processing

In a final step, we analyzed the relationship between visual and auditory temporal processing. To this end, auditory and visual parameters were submitted to bivariate consistency statistics (Cohen's Kappa). As a sensitive measure of deficits in auditory rate processing, minimum correct percentages of each subject attained at any of the three shortest ISIs of the rapid FT condition were used to predict the temporal-order thresholds in the visual domain. This analysis revealed that a significant accumulation of individuals in specific quadrants of the bivariate distribution emerged only for the control group (p < 0.05). This finding is illustrated in Figure 3: None of the controls demonstrated both low auditory accuracy (i.e., ≤ 75% correct) and high visual thresholds (i.e., ≥ 8 ms SOA), leaving the lower right quadrant empty of control participants. Children with dyslexia in contrast were scattered over the entire range in both tasks, showing no significant intermodal association.

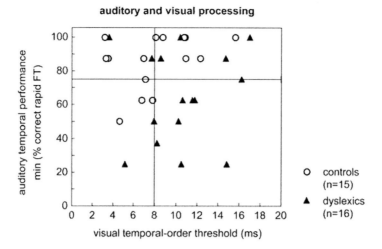

Figure 3. Auditory temporal performance in relation to visual temporal-order thresholds for controls (open circles) and dyslexics (filled triangles). 'Min (% correct rapid FT)' denotes minimum correct percentages attained at any of the three shortest ISIs of the rapid FT condition. Low visual thresholds reflect superior performance. Solid lines indicate cut-off scores for high auditory accuracy (> 75%) and low visual thresholds (< 8 ms).

Comparison of Age Groups

Data reported so far show that 11 year-old dyslexic children exhibited elevated visual temporal-order thresholds relative to controls. This is in contrast to what was observed previously in 13-year-olds (Heim et al., 2001). In this older group of participants, no significant effect of diagnosis was observed in terms of visual temporal-order thresholds. This indicated that both the dyslexics (mean = 8.87, SD = 5.54) and controls (mean = 9.93, SD = 4.37) managed the visual task without difficulty and equally well.

In both age groups, we identified two subgroups of dyslexic children in the auditory domain: One group benefited from prolonged presentation of syllables in that performance increased as a function of consonant duration (poor perceivers). The other group did not show such benefit, but scored high across formant transition lengths (good perceivers). The young sample comprised 10 poor perceivers and 6 good perceivers. In older participants, the ratio appeared reversed (see Figure 4) being characterized by 8 poor and 14 good perceivers. However, this difference between age groups did not reach statistical significance. Although samples are small and issues of statistical power cannot be completely ruled out, our results suggest that for the task used here, a certain proportion of diagnosed cases in each age group exhibit impaired discrimination of short duration stop-consonant syllables.

When comparing age groups, both younger dyslexic participants and older controls demonstrated no relationship between auditory accuracy and visual thresholds (see Figures 3 and 5). Data collected with older controls showed good auditory rate processing across the entire range of visual thresholds. As described earlier, young children with dyslexia showed a similar pattern with overall decreased accuracy in the auditory and visual tasks. In contrast, significant relationships were found in the younger control and older dyslexic group (see Figures 3 and 5). None of the younger controls and none of the older dyslexics performed poorly in both modalities, leading to an exponential pattern of the bivariate distribution function. In particular, the latter group of affected children contained a significant subset of individuals scoring low in the auditory discrimination task, but high in visual temporal processing performance.

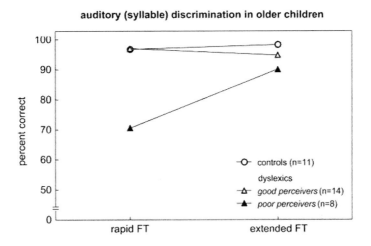

Figure 4. Percent correct responses in the auditory syllable-discrimination task for older controls (open circles) and older dyslexic children (Heim et al., 2001). As in the younger age group, dyslexics were considered good (open triangles) or poor (filled triangles) perceivers according to their discrimination accuracy in the three shortest ISIs of the rapid FT condition.

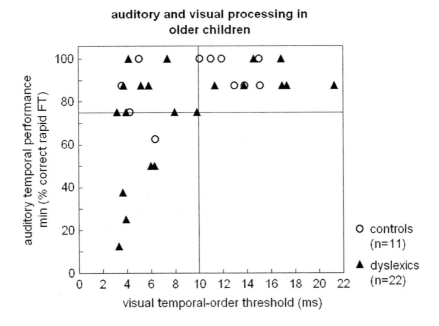

Figure 5. Auditory temporal performance in relation to visual temporal-order thresholds for the older age group (Heim et al., 2001). Controls are marked by open circles, dyslexics by filled triangles. 'Min (% correct rapid FT)' denotes minimum correct percentages attained at any ISI of the rapid FT condition. Low visual thresholds reflect superior performance. Solid lines indicate cut-off scores for high auditory accuracy (> 75%) and low visual thresholds (< 10 ms).

DISCUSSION

We observed differential changes in the correlation between auditory and visual parameters of rate processing as a function of age. In dyslexia, the relationship increased with age, whereas normal literates' panmodal associations showed a decrease over the same time scale. This pattern has several implications in light of the studies reviewed earlier in the chapter. One hypothesis considered capitalizes on the possibility of a developmental shift that mediates the outcome in pansensory studies of rate processing.

Recent work suggests that age and maturation moderate perceptual skills in the auditory modality of language-learning impaired individuals (Bishop and McArthur 2004; Hautus, Setchell, Waldie, and Kirk, 2003; Wright and Zecker, 2004). Benasich and colleagues (Benasich et al., 2006; Benasich and Leevers, 2003; Benasich and Tallal, 2002) reported that auditory rate processing abilities in infants differed as a function of family history for language impairment and were predictive of later language outcome. This has been demonstrated by using behavioral and electrocortical paradigms. Infants were tested at 7.5 months and prospectively followed through 36 months. At the first session, infants born to families with affected first-degree relatives showed significantly elevated thresholds for auditory rate processing compared to controls with no family risk of language disorders. Follow-up measures indicated that the ability to discriminate rapidly occurring sound changes was the best predictor of expressive and receptive language at 12, 16, and 24 months. At age 36 months, rate processing thresholds and being male jointly predicted about 40% of the variance in language status (Benasich and Tallal, 2002). On the neural level, 6-month-olds at risk for language-based learning disabilities were characterized by a mitigated change-detection response following a delayed negative wave in the event-related potential to tones presented in rapid succession. Across risk groups, the amplitude and latency of the negative wave were inversely correlated with indices of expressive and receptive language abilities at 24 months of age (Benasich et al., 2006).

Bishop and McArthur (2004) reported complementary results in adolescents with SLI. While diagnosed subjects and controls did not differ in an auditory task, all of the SLI participants showed aberrant electrocortical responses to the same set of stimuli. This might reflect compensatory coping mechanisms, which enable participants at an older age to achieve average performance scores at the cost of greater effort on a neural level.

Meyler and Breznitz (2005) used audio-visual stimuli in rapid succession to study intra- and cross-modal temporal processing in an adult sample. These researchers observed a marked deficit in dyslexia for fast processing of beeps on the level of overt behavior, as indexed by reaction time and accuracy measures. A developmental perspective on data in the visual domain yields a different picture. There was no evidence of a difference in signal detection accuracy as measured with d', when comparing normal and dyslexic adult readers in terms of their performance with light flashes. Although Meyler and Breznitz' task can be considered a gap detection paradigm, it involved evaluation of rhythmic structure in the visual or auditory scene, and thus may be regarded more difficult, compared with simple gap detection.

In the present data set, the difference between age groups in the visual modality suggests a developmental shift, which reflects a decrease of an initial deficit across time. Based on the distribution of visual temporal-order thresholds in both younger and older dyslexic children, task difficulty as a main determinant of this finding can be ruled out. In contrast, the auditory task might have been too easy for the controls and some of the older dyslexics. Auditory accuracy therefore might be compromised by a ceiling effect. It is important for future work to select tasks that are sensitive to different aspects of temporal processing and, at the same time, are appropriate in terms of difficulty with respect to the age group studied. Given the differences between behavioral and electrocortical parameters of rapid processing outlined above, we also recommend that a multivariate approach should be used to further examine this research question (Bishop and McArthur, 2004). In particular, measures that are sensitive to rapidly changing cortical dynamics with sufficient spatial resolution are essential to ensure coverage of the relevant process (Heim and Keil, 2004). Studies using magnetoencephalography, for instance, have pointed to distinct spatio-temporal anomalies in the processing of the stop consonant-vowel syllable /ba/ in children and adults having dyslexia (Heim, Eulitz, and Elbert, 2003a,b). This difference in the functional neuroanatomy was localized in right-hemispheric auditory cortex and occurred around 100 ms post-syllable onset, suggesting an early locus of the problem. Our data also strongly suggest that the subtype profile of a given sample needs to be taken into account. Indeed, the population under consideration represents a heterogeneous group of individuals on the symptom level, and on the level of neurocognitive markers of the condition.

To complete, the relationship between visual and auditory temporal processing in dyslexia across the two age groups can be described as follows: While younger dyslexic children may have deficits in both modalities, older dyslexics may not show co-occurrence of visual and auditory impairments.

CONCLUSION

Subjects' age has been discussed as one factor mediating performance in cross-modal rate processing, possibly leading to mixed findings in dyslexia. In particular, the developmental trajectory may be crucial for the understanding of group differences as observed in previous research. Our results indicate that a temporal dysfunction in the visual modality disappears through development (see Di Lollo et al., 1983; Tallal et al., 1981), whereas auditory problems are still detectable in adolescence. Thus, chronological age is a putative candidate for modulating panmodal temporal deficits in dyslexia. This in turn is an important impulse for ongoing and future prospective longitudinal studies examining perceptual and language processes as a function of family history for language-based learning impairments (Benasich and Leevers, 2003; Lyytinen et al., 2004).

ACKNOWLEDGEMENTS

The present study was supported by grants from the German Research Council (Deutsche Forschungsgemeinschaft). We are grateful to Robert B. Freeman, Jr. for providing the software of the visual task. Special thanks to the children who volunteered their time to participate in this study, as well as to the parents for their co-operation.

REFERENCES

Benasich, A., Choudhury, N., Friedman, J., Realpe-Bonilla, T., Chojnowska, C., and Gou, Z. (2006). The infant as a prelinguistic model for language learning impairments: Predicting from event-related potentials to behavior. *Neuropsychologia, 44,* 396–411.

Benasich, A., and Leevers, H. (2003). Processing of rapidly presented auditory cues in infancy: Implications for later language development. In H. Hayne and J. Fagen (Eds.), *Progress in infancy research* (Vol. 3, pp. 245–288). Mahwah, NJ: Erlbaum.

Benasich, A., and Tallal, P. (2002). Infant discrimination of rapid auditory cues predicts later language impairment. *Behavioural Brain Research, 136,* 31–49.

Bishop, D., Carlyon, R., Deeks, J., and Bishop, S. (1999). Auditory temporal processing impairment: Neither necessary nor sufficient for causing language impairment in children. *Journal of Speech, Language, and Hearing Research, 42,* 1295–1310.

Bishop, D., and McArthur, G. (2004). Immature cortical responses to auditory stimuli in specific language impairment: Evidence from ERPs to rapid tone sequences. *Developmental Science, 7,* F11–F18.

Byrne, B. (1981). Deficient syntactic control in poor readers: Is a weak phonetic memory code responsible? *Applied Psycholinguistics, 2,* 201–212.

Conlon, E., Sanders, M., and Zapart, S. (2004). Temporal processing in poor adult readers. *Neuropsychologia, 42,* 142–157.

Di Lollo, V., Hanson, D., and McIntyre, J. (1983). Initial stages of visual information processing in dyslexia. *Journal of Experimental Psychology/Human Perception and Performance, 9,* 923–935.

Diesch, E. (1997). SpeechLab: PC software for digital speech signal processing. *Behavior Research Methods, Instruments, and Computers, 29,* 302.

Dilling, H., Mombour, W., Schmidt, M. (1991). *International Classification of Mental Diseases, ICD-10* (German edition). Bern: Huber.

Farmer, M., and Klein, R. (1993). Auditory and visual temporal processing in dyslexic and normal readers. *Annals of the New York Academy of Sciences, 682,* 339–341.

Farmer, M., and Klein, R. (1995). The evidence for a temporal processing deficit linked to dyslexia: A review. *Psychonomic Bulletin and Review, 2,* 460–493.

Fitch, R., and Tallal, P. (2003). Neural mechanisms of language-based learning impairments: Insights from human populations and animal models. *Behavioral and Cognitive Neuroscience Reviews, 2,* 155–178.

Goswami, U. (2000). Phonological representations, reading development and dyslexia: Towards a cross-linguistic theoretical framework. *Dyslexia, 6,* 133–151.

Grissemann, H. (1998). *Zürcher Lesetest (ZLT)*. Bern: Huber.

Grund, M., Haug, G., and Naumann, C. (1994). *Diagnostischer Rechtschreibtest für 4. Klassen (DRT 4)*. Weinheim: Beltz.

Grund, M., Haug, G., and Naumann, C. (1995). *Diagnostischer Rechtschreibtest für 5. Klassen (DRT 5)*. Weinheim: Beltz.

Hari, R., and Kiesilä, P. (1996). Deficit of temporal auditory processing in dyslexic adults. *Neuroscience Letters, 205,* 138–140.

Hautus, M., Setchell, G., Waldie, K., and Kirk, I. (2003). Age-related improvements in auditory temporal resolution in reading-impaired children. *Dyslexia, 9,* 37–45.

Heim, S., Eulitz, C., and Elbert, T. (2003a). Altered hemispheric asymmetry of auditory N100m in adults with developmental dyslexia. *Neuroreport, 14,* 501–504.

Heim, S., Eulitz, C., and Elbert, T. (2003b). Altered hemispheric asymmetry of auditory P100m in dyslexia. *European Journal of Neuroscience, 17,* 1715–1722.

Heim, S., Freeman, R., Jr., Eulitz, C., and Elbert, T. (2001). Auditory temporal processing deficit in dyslexia is associated with enhanced sensitivity in the visual modality. *Neuroreport, 12,* 507–510.

Heim, S., and Keil, A. (2004). Large-scale neural correlates of developmental dyslexia. *European Child and Adolescent Psychiatry, 13,* 125–140.

Heller, K., Kratzmeier, H., and Lengfelder, A. (1998). *Raven-Matrizen-Test, Standard Progressive Matrices (SPM).* German adaptation. Göttingen: Beltz.

Joanisse, M., Manis, F., Keating, P., and Seidenberg, M. (2000). Language deficits in dyslexic children: Speech perception, phonology, and morphology. *Journal of Experimental Child Psychology, 77,* 30–60.

Lyytinen, H., Ahonen, T., Eklund, K., Guttorm, T., Kulju, P., Laakso, M., et al. (2004). Early development of children at familial risk for dyslexia: Follow-up from birth to school age. *Dyslexia, 10,* 146–178.

McAnally, K., and Stein, J. (1996). Auditory temporal coding in dyslexia. *Proceedings of the Royal Society of London. Series B, Biological Sciences, 263,* 961–965.

Merzenich, M., Jenkins, W., Johnston, P., Schreiner, C., Miller, S., and Tallal, P. (1996). Temporal processing deficits of language-learning impaired children ameliorated by training. *Science, 271,* 77–81.

Meyler, A., and Breznitz, Z. (2005). Visual, auditory and cross-modal processing of linguistic and nonlinguistic temporal patterns among adult dyslexic readers. *Dyslexia, 11,* 93–115.

Müller, R. (1997). *Diagnostischer Rechtschreibtest für 3. Klassen (DRT 3).* Weinheim: Beltz.

Newsome, W., and Paré, E. (1988). A selective impairment of motion perception following lesions of the middle temporal visual area (MT). *Journal of Neuroscience, 8,* 2201–2211.

Protopapas, A., Ahissar, M., and Merzenich, M. (1997). Auditory processing is related to reading ability. *Journal of the Acoustical Society of America, 102,* 3188.

Ramus, F. (2003). Developmental dyslexia: Specific phonological deficit or general sensorimotor dysfunction? *Current Opinion in Neurobiology, 13,* 212–218.

Rathenow, P., Laupenmühlen, D., and Vöge, J. (1981). *Westermann Rechtschreibtest 6+ (WRT 6+).* Braunschweig: Westermann.

Shapley, R. (1990). Visual sensitivity and parallel retinocortical channels. *Annual Review of Psychology, 41,* 635–658.

Snowling, M. (2000). *Dyslexia* (2nd edition). Malden, MA: Blackwell.

Stark, R., Bernstein, L., Condino, R., Bender, M., Tallal, P., and Catts, H. (1984). Four-year follow-up study of language impaired children. *Annals of Dyslexia, 34,* 49–68.

Talcott, J., Hansen, P., Assoku, E., and Stein, J. (2000). Visual motion sensitivity in dyslexia: Evidence for temporal and energy integration deficits. *Neuropsychologia, 38,* 935–943.

Tallal, P. (1980). Auditory temporal perception, phonics, and reading disabilities in children. *Brain and Language, 9,* 182–198.

Tallal, P., Miller, S., Bedi, G., Byma, G., Wang, X., Nagarajan, S., et al. (1996). Language comprehension in language-learning impaired children improved with acoustically modified speech. *Science, 271,* 81–84.

Tallal, P., and Piercy, M. (1973a). Defects of non-verbal auditory perception in children with developmental aphasia. *Nature, 241,* 468–469.

Tallal, P., and Piercy, M. (1973b). Developmental aphasia: Impaired rate of non-verbal processing as a function of sensory modality. *Neuropsychologia, 11,* 389–398.

Tallal, P., and Piercy, M. (1974). Developmental aphasia: Rate of auditory processing and selective impairment of consonant perception. *Neuropsychologia, 12,* 83–93.

Tallal, P., and Piercy, M. (1975). Developmental aphasia: The perception of brief vowels and extended stop consonants. *Neuropsychologia, 13,* 69–74.

Tallal, P., Stark, R., Kallman, C., and Mellits, D. (1981). A reexamination of some nonverbal perceptual abilities of language-impaired and normal children as a function of age and sensory modality. *Journal of Speech and Hearing Research, 24,* 351–357.

Temple, E., Deutsch, G., Poldrack, R., Miller, S., Tallal, P., Merzenich, M., et al. (2003). Neural deficits in children with dyslexia ameliorated by behavioral remediation: Evidence from functional MRI. *Proceedings of the National Academy of Sciences, USA, 100,* 2860–2865.

Tomblin, J., Zhang, X., Buckwalter, P., and Catts, H. (2000). The association of reading disability, behavioral disorders, and language impairment among second-grade children. *Journal of Child Psychology and Psychiatry, 41,* 473–482.

Van Ingelghem, M., van Wieringen, A., Wouters, J., Vandenbussche, E., Onghena, P., and Ghesquière, P. (2001). Psychophysical evidence for a general temporal processing deficit in children with dyslexia. *Neuroreport, 12,* 3603–3607.

Wilmer, J., Richardson, A., Chen, Y., and Stein, J. (2004). Two visual motion processing deficits in developmental dyslexia associated with different reading skills deficits. *Journal of Cognitive Neuroscience, 16,* 528–540.

Witton, C., Talcott, J., Hansen, P., Richardson, A., Griffiths, T., Rees, A., et al. (1998). Sensitivity to dynamic auditory and visual stimuli predicts nonword reading ability in both dyslexic and normal readers. *Current Biology, 8,* 791–797.

Wright, B., and Zecker, S. (2004). Learning problems, delayed development, and puberty. *Proceedings of the National Academy of Sciences, USA, 101,* 9942–9946.

In: Dyslexia in Children: New Research
Editor: Christopher B. Hayes, pp. 79-91

ISBN 1-59454-969-9
© 2006 Nova Science Publishers, Inc.

Chapter 4

READING ERRORS IN YOUNG ADULTS WITH VERMIS OR CEREBELLAR HEMISPHERIC LESIONS

Rita Moretti*, Paola Torre and Rodolfo M. Antonello
Department of Internal Medicine and Clinical Neurology, UCO of Clinical Neurology ,
Cognitive Disturbances Section, University of Trieste

ABSTRACT

Some evidence associates dyslexia, both developmental and acquired, with binocular instability, reduced amplitude of accomodation and reduced contrast sensitivity for both low spatial frequencies and uniform field flicker. If vision plays a dominant role in the guidance of movements, cerebellar lesions produce profound deficits in visuomotor control, considering that visual information is integrated in lobule VIc and VII of the caudal vermis important for the control of both smooth pursuit and target-directed saccades. Considering these perspectives, we studied 5 young patients with selective vermian/paravermian lesions, , and 5 young adults with selective hemispheric cerebellar lesion, who before did never complain reading troubles, in order to detect eventual difficulties or abnormalities in reading process. We have compared the results to those obtained by a group of normal volunteers. We suggest that only vermian patients (and not those with hemispheric lesions) respond imperfectly to normal controlling influences exerted by the vermis region on the SC and the pontine nuclei; therefore, this may cause inappropriate eye positioning sufficient to decrease the ability of reading. In particular, we hypothesize that vermian lesions produce a defective control of saccadic movements, fundamental for the execution of the reading task.

Key words: young, cerebellum, dyslexia, reading, visual input, binocular stability.

A written language is a cultural creation and the emergence of a written language is a function of social-cultural phenomena. Mastery of the written language typically requires

* Corresponding Author: Rita Moretti, Department of Internal Medicine and Clinical Neurology, UCO of Clinical Neurology University of Trieste, Ospedale di Cattinara, Strada di Fiume 447, 34149 TRIESTE, Italy; phone 0039-040-3994321; fax: 0039-040-910861; e-mail: moretti@univ.trieste.it

work and a level of explicit effort, which is not required for normal language acquisition or visual maturation. Thus, reading is one of the most learned competencies in humans. That is the main reason for the finding that very different brain regions are involved in the control of reading operations.

The results of neuroimaging studies converge to reveal a set of areas active during word-reading, including left-lateralized regions in occipital and occipital-temporal cortex, the left frontal operculum, bilateral regions within primary motor cortex, the superior and middle temporal cortex, the medial regions in the supplementary motor area, the anterior cyngulate gyrus and the cerebellum (Fiez and Petersen, 1998).

Dyslexia is an operationally defined condition (or group of conditions) and it appears when the automatic mechanism of word identification during reading is impaired; dyslexics are characterized mainly by difficulty with learning to read and by their inability to achieve expected reading levels.

Acquired dyslexia (usually defined alexia) occur in adulthood, or better said, in a brain which has learned normally prior to the insult, to read. Alexia may develop as a consequence of a lesion of the Wernicke's or Broca's areas or most prominently of the angular gyrus, in association with selective lesions of cuneate, fusiform, lingualis and calcarine gyri, and even with lateral geniculate lesion. Patients initially cannot read at all; as they recover, they learn to read letter by letter, spelling out words laboriously. Patients cannot read words at glance, as skilled readers can do. By contrast, they quickly understand words spelled orally ad they can spell normally.

On the other hand, in the restricted definition of developmental dyslexia, the reading difficulty may be part of a more generalized disturbance of sensory motor functions; in fact, dyslexics manifest other difficulties, such as an impairment of long and short term memory, of orientation, of equilibrium, and of time management. Other common characteristics of dyslexics like left/right confusion or sequencing problems, should be included in the definition. In fact, most experts in the field agreed that dyslexia represents a true behavioral anomaly, rather than simply an extreme example of normal variation in reading competencies (Galaburda, 2002).

Whatever the contributions of other systems and processes, there is now a strong consensus among investigators in the field that the central difficulty in dyslexia reflects a deficiency within the phonologic module, which is engaged in processing the sounds of speech (Share and Stanovich, 1995).

Although dyslexic individuals exhibit some abnormalities of visual processing, (Demb et al., 1997), a strong consensus has emerged, which proposes that a central difficulty in dyslexia is the processing of speech sounds, known as phonological processing (Grigorenko, 2001). According to the phonologic deficit hypothesis, people with dyslexia have difficulty developing an awareness that words, both written and spoken, can be broken down into smaller units of sound and that, in fact, the letters constituting the printed word represent the sounds heard in the spoken word. There is abundant evidence that a deficit in phonological analysis is related to difficulties in learning to read: phonologic measures predict later reading achievement (Torgesen et al., 1994); deficits in phonologic awareness (i.e. awareness that words can be broken down into smaller segments of sound) consistently distinguish children with dyslexia from those who are not reading-impaired (Stanovich and Siegel, 1992); phonologic deficits persist into adulthood; and instruction in phonological awareness promotes the acquisition of reading skills (Lefly and Pennington, 1991; Shaywitz, 1998).

In dyslexia, a deficit at the level of the phonologic module impairs the ability to segment the written word into its underlying phonologic elements. As a result, the reader experiences difficulty, first in decoding the word and then in identifying it. The phonologic deficit is domain-specific; that is, it is independent of other nonphonologic abilities. According to the model, a circumscribed deficit in a lower-order linguistic (phonologic) function blocks access to higher-order processes and to the ability to draw meaning from text.

Nevertheless, many theories of dyslexia have been proposed, apart from the phonological alterations, and these hypothesis are based on micro-alterations of the visual system, and the disruption of the temporal processing of stimuli within these systems. Different anatomical, electrophysiological and brain-imaging studies (Stein and Walsh, 1997) have begun to take into account the complaint of many dyslexics (both developmental and acquired): small letters appear to blur and move around when they are trying to read. The defect does not seem to arise from a single visual relay but, as mentioned above, from abnormalities of the magnocellular component of the visual system, specialized for processing fast temporal information and for managing control of eye movements.

On these bases, abundant evidence correlates dyslexia to binocular instability (dyslexics make fewer visual errors, if they read with only one eye; Cornelissen et al, 1998), reduced amplitude of accomodation and reduced contrast sensitivity for both low spatial frequencies and uniform field flicker (Evans et al., 1996). On the contrary, Skottun (2000) has criticized these points, and in a vast review concluded that although there are clearly studies consistent with a magnocellular deficit, these studies are outnumbered both by studies that have found no deficits, and by studies that have found deficits that are incompatible with magnicellular impairment.

The most salient aspects of the criticisms induced is that magnocellular neurons respond most vigorously to coarse (i.e. low spatial frequency) patterns when these undergo rapid temporal changes (such as in the case of rapidly moving stimuli) (Skottun, 2000 B). It is not clear how a defect in the reading of printed characters, that are stationary and that are distinguishable mainly on the basis of fine details, could be the result of a magnocellular deficit, which is related to perception of movement stimuli. Other workers, from a different speculative point of view, have also derived intervention of visual perception and peripheral vision in explication of dyslexia (Geiger and Lettvin, 1987; Geiger and Lettvin, 1994). Their work found that dyslexics and normal readers differ in relation to foveal and peripheral vision. Directly related to the "peripheral masking,", their experiments showed that in dyslexics, there is an interaction between foveal and peripheral vision that degrades the ability to read in foveal field. Normal reading seems to involve a learned strategy for suppressing or masking information away from the fovea. Hence, the Form-Resolving Field (FRF) of the normal readers is narrow (foveal) and symmetrical (binocular), with the best recognition of letter in and immediately near the center of gaze.

Recognition of individual letters degrades as the angular distance from the gaze decreases. In contrast, the FRF of dyslexic subjects is wider, but not so precise in the direction of reading. By this hypothesis, it is possible to explain the inability to associate the clients names with details of their cases, difficulties in verb generation tasks and in error detection tasks, as a consequence of a right cerebellar ischemia (Fiez et al., 1994; Stein and Glickstein, 1992, Moretti et al., 2003).

Therefore, some evidence associates dyslexia, both developmental and acquired, with binocular instability, reduced amplitude of accomodation and reduced contrast sensitivity for both low spatial frequencies and uniform field flicker (Cornelissen *et al.*, 1998). In humans, most movements are either triggered or guided by visual stimuli.

If vision plays a dominant role in the guidance of movements, cerebellar lesions produce profound deficits in visuomotor control, considering that visual information is integrated in lobule VIc and VII of the caudal vermis important for the control of both smooth pursuit and target-directed saccades (Buttner *et al.*, 1986; Moretti et al. 2002).

Considering these perspectives, we studied 5 young patients with selective vermian/paravermian lesions, , and 5 young adults with selective hemispheric cerebellar lesion, who before did never complain reading troubles, in order to detect eventual difficulties or abnormalities in reading process. We have compared the results to those obtained by a group of normal volunteers.

SUBJECTS AND METHODS

We studied 5 right-handed patients who suffered from a vermian/paravermian tumour, and 5 right-handed patients who suffered from hemispheric cerebellar tumour, demonstrated by NMR, and histological examination.

Patients Case History

1. R.V. (18 year -old woman) presented with a 7 months history of general slowing up, with unsteadiness of gait; on neurological examination, she demonstrated slight dysmetria in finger to finger tasks. She obtained a score of 14/35 in the ataxia score evaluation; no signs of dysarthria emerged (Klockgether et al., 1990). Magnetic resonance imaging revealed the presence of an arachnoidal cyst of the vermis.

2. S.D. (27 year -old woman) presented with a 3 months history of unsteadiness of gait; on neurological examination, she demonstrated slight dysmetria in finger to finger tasks. She obtained a score of 23/35 in the ataxia score evaluation; no signs of dysarthria emerged (Klockgether et al., 1990). Magnetic resonance imaging revealed the presence of an arachnoidal cyst of the vermis, located near the periquadrigemellar fossa.

3. F.D. (19 year -old woman) presented with a 6 months history of unsteadiness of gait and diplopia on right-extreme lateral gaze; on neurological examination, she demonstrated slight dysmetria, a modest gait unsteadiness. She obtained a score of 14/35 in the ataxia score evaluation; no signs of dysarthria emerged (Klockgether et al., 1990). Magnetic resonance imaging revealed the presence of a hypervascularized lesion of the vermis, with slight surrounding oedema, which appeared to be a hemangioma, at histological specimen.

4. E.F. (22 year -old woman) presented with a 1 month history of vertigos, unsteadiness of gait, severe headache and dysmetria; on neurological examination, she demonstrated an evident dysmetria in finger to finger tasks, gait ataxia, and disdiadochokinesia. She obtained a score of 30/35 in the ataxia score evaluation; very modest signs of dysarthria emerged (1/5) (Klockgether et al., 1990). Magnetic resonance imaging revealed the presence of a hyperintense lesion of the vermis, with concomitant and diffuse

perilesional oedema, which appears to be an astrocytoma (confirmed at histology as a grade 2).

5. F.P. (21 year –old man) presented with a 9 months history of violent headache, nausea and vomiting, with unsteadiness of gait and disequilibrium; on neurological examination, he demonstrated slight dysmetria in finger to finger tasks and disdiadochokinesia. He obtained a score of 15/35 in the ataxia score evaluation; no signs of dysarthria emerged (Klockgether et al., 1990). Magnetic resonance imaging revealed the presence of an arachnoidal cyst of the vermis, which lays near the periquadrigemellar cysterna, without surrounding oedema.

6. W.M. (19 year -old woman) presented with a 7 months history of general slowing up, with unsteadiness of gait, and violent headache; on neurological examination, she demonstrated slight dysmetria in finger to finger tasks. She obtained a score of 19/35 in the ataxia score evaluation; modest signs of dysarthria emerged (2/5)(Klockgether et al., 1990). Magnetic resonance imaging revealed the presence of an arachnoidal cyst of the right cerebellar hemisphere.

7. B.B. (20 year -old woman) presented with a 2 months history of unsteadiness of gait, particularly evident while playing tennis, headache and vomiting; on neurological examination, she demonstrated slight dysmetria in finger to finger tasks and a modest gait ataxia (18/35 in the ataxia score evaluation); no signs of dysarthria emerged (Klockgether et al., 1990). Magnetic resonance imaging revealed the presence of an arachnoidal cyst of the left hemisphere of the cerebellum.

8. A.P. (26 year -old woman) presented with a 8 months history of slight unsteadiness of gait, modest dysarthria, headache and nausea for two weeks; on neurological examination, she demonstrated slight dysmetria in finger to finger tasks, a modest gait ataxia and unsteadiness (21/35 in the ataxia score evaluation), and a slight dysarthria emerged (2/5) (Klockgether et al., 1990). Magnetic resonance imaging revealed the presence of a hypervascularized lesion of the right cerebellar hemisphere, with slight surrounding oedema, which appeared to be a hemangioblastoma, at histological specimen.

9. L.S. (29 year -old woman) presented with a 3 months history of dizziness, dysarthria, dysmetria, headache and nausea; on neurological examination, she demonstrated an evident dysmetria in finger to finger tasks, hypotonia of the right hemisoma, and disdiadochokinesia. She obtained a score of 23/35 in the ataxia score evaluation; mild signs of dysarthria emerged (1/5) (Klockgether et al., 1990). Magnetic resonance imaging revealed the presence of a hyperintense lesion, with concomitant and diffuse perilesional oedema, which appears to be an astrocytoma (confirmed at histology as a grade 3) of the right cerebellar hemisphere.

10. G.C (19 year -old woman) presented with a 7 months history of unsteadiness of gait and diplopia on left-extreme lateral gaze; on neurological examination, she demonstrated slight dysmetria, a modest gait unsteadiness. She obtained a score of 19/35 in the ataxia score evaluation; no signs of dysarthria emerged (Klockgether et al., 1990). Magnetic resonance imaging revealed the presence of a hypervascularized lesion of the left hemisphere of the cerebellum, with slight surrounding oedema, which appeared to be a hemangioblastoma, at histological specimen.

No patients complained for reading alterations, before the admission.

For all the patients we obtained neuroimaging, a complete neurological observation, and an oculomotor evaluation. Eye movements were recorded by means of an infrared pupil reflection system (AMTech ET3 eye tracking system). This enables measuring movements in both horizontal and vertical directions for each eye. The system has an absolute accuracy of $0.25°$. Saccadic eye movements were measured in a single target and in a sequential target task. The standard deviations of the saccadic reaction times and the amount of late saccades were compared to normal control. We evaluated gain in pursuit movements, tested at 0.1, 0.2, 0.3 and 0.4 Hz., as well as accuracy of both fixed and random saccadic movements, and number of regressive movements and duration of fixations.

Informed consent was obtained from all the subjects prior to the study and the study has been approved by Ethical Local Committee.

Both patients and controls, underwent to handedness test of Briggs and Nebes (1975), to an evaluation of bucco-facial apraxia and of visual gnosia (Spinnler and Tognoni, 1987). Their intelligence capabilities was evaluated by Raven Standard Progressive Matrices (Valseschini and Del Ton., 1994). They underwent to the Bilingual Aphasia Test (BAT) (Paradis and Canzanella, 1990).

As far as the reading capacities are concerned, all subjects were asked to read 70 commonly used words in the Italian language and 70 non-words. Words and non-words varied along visual-linguistic dimensions, such as length (6-10 letters) and for words, frequency (medium-high frequency in Italian language). Words and non-words were presented for seven seconds each, in upper case letters, centred on a high resolution computer monitor. Before starting with these tests, subjects were instructed to read single letters, presented on the same monitor, to make them confident with the system: all the letters were correctly recognised by the patients of both groups and by the control match. The subjects were then asked to read a text obtained from the BAT (59 words) (Paradis and Canzanella, 1990) and ten sentences (for a total of 67 words) (Paradis and Canzanella, 1990).

All the material read by the subjects was recorded on audio-tape and subsequently analysed; two trained neurologists, PT and RM, whose professional interests focused on cognition, listened separately the tape recordings; accuracy and inter-rate reliability is quite high (kappa=0.89, p<0.01). We did not take into account doubt situations or imprecision mainly due to tape-recording defects. In case of permanent doubts, after comparison, a discussion was effectuated and final decision derived from a mutual consensus.

RESULTS

All the subjects, patients and controls, were right-handed (+22 at the test of Briggs and Nebes, 1975); there were no signs of bucco-facial apraxia and of visual agnosia (Spinnler and Tognoni, 1987). Their average educational levels was of 12 + 1.45 years, and all of them, both patients and controls, considered themselves as expert readers, by means of daily reading almost of books, newspapers and magazines.

There was a different average score for dysarthria in the two groups: the mean Klochgether score was 0.6 ± 0.1 (Klockgether et al., 1990).

Their intelligence capabilities were considered on the average values of the 79th-86th percentile (Valseschini and Del Ton., 1994). No signs of language alteration (considering morphology and syntax), and no signs of disruption of language comprehension, according to the Bilingual Aphasia Test (BAT) (Paradis and Canzanella, 1990) can be detected in all the subjects.

Statistical analysis was performed with the Statistical Package for the Social Sciences (SPSS version 10.0) For comparisons between the two groups a t-test of Student and analysis of variance (ANOVA) were used as appropriate. Spearmann rank correlation analysis has been employed. Errors rates in the different conditions (words, non words, sentences and text) have been compared using ANOVA, adjusted for group and type of mistakes.

The total number of items presented to all the subjects was 266 (words/non-words/ words in the sentences and in the text).

Patients with cerebellar vermis lesions produced, in all the four reading tasks, a mean number of 87.58 ± 11.23 mistakes. Mistakes can be divided as follows: they made 19.32 ± 2.33 mistakes in words-reading task, 20.59 ± 2.67 mistakes in non words-reading task, 26.11 ± 1.34 mistakes in the sentences reading task, and 20.65 ± 3.89 mistakes in the text reading task.

Patients with cerebellar hemispheric lesions produced, in all the four reading tasks, a mean number of 32.3 ± 5.78 mistakes. Mistakes can be divided as follows: they made 10.85 ± 1.34 mistakes in words-reading task, 8.47 ± 0.23 mistakes in non words-reading task, 9.59 ± 1.45 mistakes in the sentences reading task, and 3.08 ± 0.56 mistakes in the text reading task.

According to a t-test, there are important differences among the number of mistakes in the two groups of cerebellar patients, as evidenced by table 1. In all the four tasks, there was a significant larger amount ($p<0.01$) of mistakes in vermis patients comparing with hemispheric cerebellar patients' corpus of mistakes.

Dysarthria has been evaluated, as previously stated, by Klockgether scale (Klockgether et al., 1990). There was a different average score for dysarthria in the two groups: the mean Klochgether score was 0.6 ± 0.1 (Klockgether et al., 1990). It was not found a correlation between reading errors and degree of cerebellar dysarthria in the two groups, considering a Spearmann rank correlation analysis.

We obtained oculomotor evaluation for all the subjects involve in the study; a set of univariate ANOVAs indicate that the amount of late saccades were increased in cerebellar vermis patients, compared to hemispheric lesions($p<0.01$), that there was a low gain in pursuit movements, tested at 0.1, 0.2, 0.3 and 0.4 Hz. Compared to hemispheric lesions ($p<0.01$), that there was an higher percentage of correction of initial undershooting with a second forward saccade in cerebellar vermis patients ($p<0.001$), and lastly that there is an increased number of regressive movements, with longer time of fixations (more than 294 ± 32.45 ms) ($p<0.001$) when compared to normal subjects. A positive correlation has been found between the amount of late saccades and the total number of reading mistakes in vermis patients ($p<0.01$), and between the low gain of pursuits and reading mistakes ($p<0.01$) in vermis patients, considering a Spearmann rank correlation analysis.

DISCUSSION

The main finding in the present study is the clear reading difficulty among cerebellar vermian patients, which is a confirm of the two previous published studies (Moretti et al., 2002; Moretti et al., 2003).

Thus, patients, who were not dyslexic before the lesion, and who presents lesions of the vermis produced a great number of mistakes, while reading. On the contrary, patients with hemispheric cerebellar lesions presented a limited number of reading mistakes. The other difference is that vermis patients did show ocular alteration, in particular a greater amount of late saccades, a low gain in pursuit movements, a higher percentage of correction of initial undershooting with a second forward saccade, and an increased number of regressive movements, with longer time of fixations (more than 294 ± 32.45 ms) when compared to normal subjects. A positive correlation has been found between the amount of late saccades and the total number of reading mistakes in vermis patients, and between the low gain of pursuits and reading mistakes in these patients. Hemispheric cerebellar patients did not show ocular movement alterations and did not show the major problems in reading, exhibited by the vermis patients.

We argue from that point, that it is not the cerebellum per se to determine the reading alterations, but specific structures of the organ, the vermis, that is intimately cor related to the ocular stability to originate the visual problems which underline the reading alteration registered.

Visually guided eye movements, saccadic and smooth pursuit, are tightly bound to reading. The primary function of the saccadic system is to orient gaze to visual targets for foveal weaving, whereas the function of the pursuit system is to maintain visual targets within the fovea, when either the stimulus or the individual is in motion. Saccades that occur during reading place a given region of the text in foveal vision for detailed processing. It is only when the eye is relatively still in a fixation that new information is extracted from the text. The average fixation duration for skilled readers is between 200-250 ms, and the eyes typically move 7-9 character spaces with each saccade. In addition, skilled readers regress to material that they have already read about 10-15% of the time. For a given reader, there is a considerable amount of variability associated with each of the mean values and is related to the reader's cognitive processes involved in understanding of the text; readers tend to look at difficult words longer than easier words and when text processing is difficult, readers make shorter saccades and more regressions (Rayner, 1998).

Cognitive factors can affect saccadic latency and accuracy, fixation duration, frequency and density, but not their velocity. Before the eyes are launched into the ballistic flight of a saccade, computation about the location of a even single word to be fixated must be made. These computations involved cortical and subcortical brain mechanisms: the sensory information from the retina is transmitted to the nervous structures that perform motor execution. Visual feedback occurs at some point at the end of the saccade and corrections to the motor program are made through corrective saccades. Beginning and disabled readers tend to make more and longer fixations, shorter saccades and more regression than skilled readers. These facts have been known for some time and often have been used to argue that eye movements are a causative factors in poor reading and since poor readers make shorter saccades each time they move their eyes, they have smaller perceptual span than skilled readers (Rayner, 1998).

Being of such importance, ocular control is a fundamental and complex indeed mechanism. Steady gaze-holding requires a tonic level of innervation to hold the eye in eccentric positions og gaze against elastic restoring forces. Ocular motor integrators take velocity commands from the conjugate systems and mathematically integrate them to produce the necessary position commands. Then, when the eye explore the environment, a specific system has been developed, the saccade.

The key to understanding why saccades evolved is to consider the primate retina, which has a foveal (macular) region of high visual acuity, corresponding to the densest distribution of photoreceptors. When we visually search the environment, we point the fovea at features of interest, moving from one point to the next with saccades. Species lacking a fovea (such as the rabbit, which has a broad "streak" of concentrated photoreceptors) do not need to make ocular saccades, although they may make combined eye-head saccades to change the center of their visual world, as well as reflexive quick phases during body rotation (Leigh, 2005).

The ocular motoneurons receive the saccadic pulse from a group of "burst neurons" lying in the brainstem reticular formation that have extraordinary properties. Burst neurons for horizontal saccades lie in the paramedian pontine reticular formation (PPRF), and for vertical and torsional fast movements lie in the rostral interstitial nucleus of the medial longitudinal fasciculus (riMLF), in the prerubral fields of the midbrain. Burst neurons discharge vigorously (up to 1000 spikes/second in monkey) *only* during saccades; at all other times they are silent (Leigh, 2005).

Clearly, a "switch" is needed to inhibit burst neurons at all times except when a saccade must be generated. A population of "omnipause neurons" serves this function; they are active at all times *except* during saccades, when they cease discharge. Omnipause neurons lie in the nucleus raphe interpositus (RIP) in the midline of the pons, and project to burst neurons in *both* the PPRF and riMLF. One other contributor to this brainstem machine that generates saccades is "latch neurons" that inhibit the omnipause neurons until the saccade is finished and the eye is on target. Current evidence suggests that the latch neurons receive a copy of burst neurons output and, when that ceases, discharge of omnipause neurons resumes (data and literature in Leigh, 2005).

The signals to start a saccade of a specified size and direction depend on neurons with visual and executive properties that are found in the parietal and frontal eye fields and the superior colliculus, to which they project. Recent data obtained from f-MRI suggest the precise cerebro-cortical organization of visually guided saccades in humans. The findings indicate saccade-related activation in frontal cortex (Broadmann areas 4 and 6) necessary for target selection and attentive polarization, and parietal areas (Schmahmann and Pandya, 1995; Ungerleider and Mishkin, 1982).

The voluntary control of saccades concerns multiple cortical areas and parallel descending pathways. A simplified view of this pathway is that it is composed of two serial, inhibitory links: a caudate-nigral inhibition, which is phasically active, and a nigrocollicular inhibition, which is tonically active. If frontal cortex causes caudate neurons to fire, then nigro-collicular inhibition is removed, and the superior colliculus is able to activate a saccade. In addition, the subthalamic nucleus contains neurons that discharge with saccades, and excites the substantia nigra pars reticulata (SNpr), which, in turn, inhibits the superior colliculus. The basal ganglion pathway appears important for programming of saccades that will be rewarded (Leigh, 2005). The mechanism that guides the saccade to its target is more problematic for the brain, since vision is inherently slow (reaction time about 100 ms) whereas most saccades are completed within this time period. For this function, the cerebellum plays a key role. Specifically, there is evidence that both the dorsal vermis, and the fastigial nucleus to which it projects, provide feedback control of saccades. Some evidence suggests that the cerebellum achieves this through "start" and "stop" commands.

The dorsal vermis (lobules VI and VII) and the underlying posterior fastigial nucleus (FN, also called the fastigial oculomotor region or FOR) are important in the control of saccades. This includes not only amplitude (accuracy) but also dynamic characteristics (velocity, acceleration and duration) and initiation time (latency) (Honda et al., 1997). Stimulation evoked saccades on most of the electrode as it advanced through the depth of the vermis, and it was possible to map the threshold for evoking saccades along a penetration as well as to ascertain the tissue situated at stimulation points. On penetration where saccades were evoked, there was some low-threshold regions, located in fiber tracts and not in the Purkinje or other cellular layers of the cerebellar cortex. Purkinje cells in the oculomotor vermis inhibit the ipsilateral FN. The FN projects through the contralateral superior cerebellar peduncle to the pontine and medullary reticular formation on the opposite (to the FN) side. The FN normally facilitates contralaterally directed saccades, perhaps through activity on inhibitory burst neurons that normally act to help stop saccades. Thus, a lesion of the FN results in hypermetria of ipsiversive and hypometria of contraversive saccades (Robinson et al., 1993). Bilateral FN lesions produce hypermetric saccades. In the extreme case, FN lesions cause macrosaccadic oscillations, in which saccades overshoot by so much that the patient can not acquire the central fixation target (Robinson et al., 1993). Lesions in the oculomotor vermis produce similar types of defects to those in the FN. The direction of the abnormality relative to the side of the lesion, however, is opposite to that seen with FN lesions. This is due to the fact that Purkinje cells inhibit their target neurons in the cerebellar nuclei. Thus, with a unilateral lesion, contraversive saccades are hypermetric and ipsiversive saccades are hypometric. Bilateral lesions of the oculomotor vermis produce hypometric saccades (Mossman et al., 1997).

Changes in saccade latency are seen with unilateral lesions of the cerebellar vermis, being delayed toward the side to which saccades are hypometric. Lesions in the FN and oculomotor vermis can also affect saccade velocity and especially acceleration and deceleration (Robinson et al., 1993; Robinson et al., 2000). Lesions in the oculomotor vermis lead to defects in saccade learning (an inability to adjust saccade amplitude) and in pursuit learning (an inability to adjust the initial acceleration of pursuit). Thus, like the flocculus/paraflocculus, the dorsal vermis is important for various types of ocular motor learning within its own domain, the control of saccade and pursuit accuracy (Robinson et al., 2000).

Visual information conveyed by the mossy and the climbing fibers is integrated in the Purkinje cells of the cerebellar vermis (lobules V, VI, VII) (Buttner *et al.*, 1986; Crowdy *et al.*, 2000). The flocculonodular lobe and the vermis modulate the position or the velocity of the eyes with respect to the orientation of the head and of the body, enabling the subject to fixate clearly on a new target, repositioning the gaze as in the saccadic eye movements, or to fixate clearly points while moving, and in the refining of motor commands before they reach the eyes muscles (Llinàs, 1975; Riva and Giorgi, 2000).

The mossy projections to the dorsal paraflocculus and to the lobules VI and VII of the vermis (via the dorsalis-lateralis pontine nuclei -DLPN-) derived from areas 5 and 7 of the posterior parietal cortex, from the superior colliculus (SC), from the lateral geniculate nucleus (LGN), and from the pretectum. The projections from the SC to the cerebellum possess a point-to-point projection from the retina, and to it arrive impulses from the oculomotor, the neck afferents and from the Frontal Eye Fields (FEF).

What we have seen in this study partially support the previous studies on the cerebellum vermis (Moretti et al., 2002; Moretti et al., 2003). Nevertheless, the study sheds light on the differential role of the vermis in oculomotor control, when comparing with the hypthesized role of henipsheric cerebellar lesions. We suggest that only vermian patients (and not those with hemispheric lesions) respond imperfectly to normal controlling influences exerted by the vermis region on the SC and the pontine nuclei; therefore, this may cause inappropriate eye positioning sufficient to decrease the ability of reading. In particular, we hypothesize that vermian lesions produce a defective control of saccadic movements, fundamental for the execution of the reading task.

REFERENCES

Briggs GC. and Nebes RD. Patterns of hand preference in a student population. *Cortex,* 1975; 11: 230-238.

Buttner U, Boyle R., Markert G. Cerebellar control of eye movements. *Progress in Brain Research,* 1986; 64: 225-233.

Cornelissen PL., Hansen PC. Hutton JL., Evangelinou V., Stein JF. Magnocellular visual function and children's single word reading. *Vision Res.,* 1998; 38: 471-482.

Crowdy KA, Hollands MA, Ferguson IT, Marple-Horvat DE.Evidence for interactive locomotor and oculomotor deficits in cerebellar patients during visually guided stepping. *Exp. Brain Res.,* 2000; 135: 437-454.

Demb JB, Boynton GM, Heeger DJ. Brain activity in visual cortex predicts individual differences in reading performace. *Proc. Natl. Acad. Sci.* USA 1997; 94: 13363-13366.

Evans B. J., Drasdo N., Richards I. L. (1996) Dyslexia: the link with visual deficits. *Ophtalmic Physiol. Opt.,* 16: 3-10.

Fiez J. A., Petersen S. E. Neuroimaging studies of word reading. *Proc. Natl. Acad. Sci.* USA., 1998; 95: 914-921.

Fiez JA, Petersen SE, Cheney MK, Raichle ME. Impaired non-motor learning and error detection associated with cerebellar damage. *Brain* 115: 155-178, 1994.

Galaburda AM. Dyslexia: clinical and research issues. American Academy of Neurology, San Diego 2002; 2FC.002-1-29.

Geiger G., Lettvin J. Peripheral vision in persons with dyslexia. *N.Engl. J. Med.* 1987; 316: 1238-11243.

Geiger G., Lettvin JY. Dyslexic children learn a new visual strategy for reading. A controlled experiment. *Vision Res. 1994;* 34: 1223-1233.

Grigorenko EL. Developmental dyslexia: an update on genes, brains, and environments. *J. Child Psychol. Psychiatry*, 2001; 42: 91-125.

Honda M, Zee DS, Hallett M Cerebellar control of voluntary saccadic eye movements in humans: fMRI study. *Soc Neurosci Abstr.* 1997; 23: 18.

Klockgether T, Schroth G, Diener HC, Dichgans J. Idiopathic cerebellar ataxia of late onset: natural history and MRI morphology. *J. Neurol. Neurosurg Psychiatry,* 1990; 53: 297-305.

Lefly DL, Pennington BF. Spelling errors and reading fluency in compensated adult dyslexics. *Ann. Dys.*1991; 41: 143-162.

Leigh RJ. Abnormal eye movement: which genetic disorders? American Academy of Neurology, Miami, 2005; 2DS.002: 1-46.

Llinás R. The cortex of the cerebellum. *Scientific American,* 1975; 232: 56-71.

Moretti R, Bava A, Antonello RM, Torre P. Reading errors in patients with cerebellar vermis lesions. *Journal of Neurology,* 2002; 249: 461-468.

Moretti R, Torre P., Antonello RM, Cazzato G, Bava A. The cerebellum and reading process. Nova Biomedical Books, NewYork., 2003.

Mossman S, Halmagyi GM Partial ocular tilt reaction due to unilateral cerebellar lesion. *Neurology* 1997; 49: 491-493.

Paradis M., Canzanella M. The assessment of Bilingual Aphasia. *Hillsdale* (N.Y.), Lawrence Erlbaum Associates, 1990.

Rayner, K. Eye movements in reading and information processing: twenty years of research. *Psychological Bulletins* 1998, 124, 372-422.

Riva D., Giorgi C. The cerebellum contributes to higher functions during development: evidence from a series of children surgically treated for posterior fossa tumours. *Brain,* 2000; 123 (5): 1051-1061.

Robinson FR Role of the cerebellar posterior interpositus nucleus in saccades I. Effect of temporary lesions. *J Neurophysiol.* 2000; 84:1289-1302.

Robinson FR, Straube A, Fuchs AF. Role of the caudal fastigial nucleus in saccade generation. II. Effects of muscimol inactivation. *J Neurophysiol* 1993; 70:1741-1758.

Schmahmann JD, Pandya DN. Prefrontal cortex projections to the basilar pons in rhesus monkey: implications for the cerebellar contribution to higher function. *Neuroscience Letters* 1995; 199(3): 175-178.

Share DL, Stanovich KE. Cognitive processes in early reading development: accommodating individual differences into a model of acquisition. *Issues Educ Contrib Educ Psychol* 1995; 1: 1-57.

Shaywitz SE. Dyslexia. *The New England Journal of Medicine,*1998; 338 (5): 307-312.

Skottun BC. On the conflicting support for the magnocellular deficit theory of dyslexia. *Trends in Cognitive Sciences* 2000; 4 (6): 211-212.

Skottun BC. The magnocellular deficit theory of dyslexia: the evidence from contrast sensitivity. *Vision Research* 2000; 40: 111-127.

Spinnler H., Tognoni G. Standardizzazione e taratura italiana dei test neuropsicologici. *The Italian Journal of Neurological Sciences,* 1987; S 6: 23-116.

Stanovich KE, Siegel LS. Phenotypic performance profile of children with reading disabilities: a regression-based test of the phonological-core-variable difference model. *J. Educ. Psychol.*1992; 84: 364-370.

Stein, J., Walsh, V. To see but not to read; the magnocellular theory of dyslexia. *Trends in Neuroscience,*1997; 20, 147-152.

Stein, JF, Glickstein, M. Role of the cerebellum in visual guidance of movement. Physiological Review, 1992; 72, 967-1017.

Torgesen JK, Wagner RK, Rashotte CA. Longitudinal studies of phonological processing and reading. *J. Learn. Disabil.* 1994; 27: 276-286.

Ungerleider LG, Mishkin M. Two cortical visual systems. In: Ingle DJ, Goodale MA, Mansfield RJW (eds.) *Analysis of visual behavior.* Cambridge, MA: MIT Press, 1982: 549-586.

Valseschini S., Del Ton F. Le Matrici Progressive di Raven. Contributo alla taratura su 1123 Soggetti e considerazioni sulla validità e attendibilità della prova. Organizzazioni Speciali, Firenze, 1994.

In: Dyslexia in Children: New Research
Editor: Christopher B. Hayes, pp. 93-101

Chapter 5

SUBITIZING AND COUNTING BY VISUAL MEMORY IN DYSLEXIA AND DYSCALCULIA: DEVELOPMENT, DEFICITS, TRAINING AND TRANSFER

Burkhart Fischer
Brain Research Unit, Institute of Biophysics
Albert Ludwigs University, Freiburg
Hansastr. 9, D - 79104, Freiburg
Germany

ABSTRACT

Deficits in auditory or visual perception or in saccade control contribute to problems in acquiring reading and spelling. The corresponding examination of the perceptual and optomotor skills have shown developmental deficits in comparison with age matched control groups. This chapter describes the development, deficits, and training effects of a special visual function called subitizing. This function enables subjects to recognize immediately (= subito, lat.) a small number of items even when they were presented only for short periods of time.

INTRODUCTION

Deficits in auditory or visual perception or in saccade control contribute to problems in acquiring reading and spelling. The corresponding examination of the perceptual and optomotor skills have shown developmental deficits in comparison with age matched control groups (Fischer, Hartnegg, and Mokler, 2000; Fischer et al., 2000; Fischer and Hartnegg, 2004; Biscaldi, Fischer, and Hartnegg, 2000). Selective improvements of these basic skills by daily practice yielded corresponding improvements in reading and spelling (Schäffler, Sonntag, and Fischer, 2004; Fischer and Hartnegg, 2000).

This chapter describes the development, deficits, and training effects of a special visual function called subitizing. This function enables subjects to recognize immediately (= subito, lat.) a small number of items even when they were presented only for short periods of time (Mandler and Shebo, 1982; Cowan, 2001; Balakrishnan and Ashby, 1991). Short means, that the time is too short to scan and count the items by saccadic eye movements. Subito means that a counting process is not necessary because the time to recognize one or two or three items is the same. Only when the number of items increases beyond 4 the recognition of the number increases by an almost constant time for each additional item (Jensen, Reese, and Reese, 1950; Trick and Phylyshyn, 1994). This fact indicates, that an internal counting process takes place in the brain. (When we use "counting" we do not mean counting the numbers of items at all, but counting them on the basis of an internal presentation in the memory obtained by a short presentation of the items. Similarly, we will use "subitizing", when talking about the total process of finding the number of items in the task described below).

From earlier studies it is known that visual number enumeration (tested by a discrimination task) improves with age from 6 to 22 years (Trick, Enns, and Brodeur, 1996). A number of studies have shown, that subitizing is possible by young infants (Silverman and Rose, 1980) and children (Starkey and Cooper, 1980; Starkey and Cooper, 1995).

This study uses displays of items (not discrimination) to probe the ability of subitizing and counting, when the presentation time was too short to allow scanning and enumeration by saccades.

The fact, that a percentage of children has specific difficulties in dealing with numbers (dyscalculia) has been attributed to a deficits in the sense of number (Dehaene, 1999; Stanescu-Cosson et al., 2000). The hypothesis was put forward, that the basic visual capacity of subitizing was not available in these subjects, when they were supposed to develop this sense of number: the subjects learned the digits (the visual signs of numbers) and the words (the auditory signs of numbers) but they do not have a clear idea of how many items are meant.

If such a basic visual deficit was a main factor in developing the phenomenon of dyscalculia then one should be able

1. to examine this visual capacity and show the deficit directly in single subjects
2. to reduce the difficulty by daily practice and show the improvement
3. to finally show that trained subjects profit from the training when operating with numbers.

This chapter describes step by step the attempts outlined above when applied to children with problems in reading and/or spelling and in children with problems in basic arithmetic skills.

DEVELOPMENT

Before we can proceed and describe the development we need a standardized task of subitizing and number counting. The test task must be designed to allow its application in high numbers of subjects, especially in children to see the possible development during the period of life when children visit school in an age range from 7 to 17 years.

Such a standardized task, called "CountFix" (from German fix = fast) was implemented in a hand held box with an LCD-display (2,5cm x 6cm in size) and an array of digit keys. Different numbers of items (small circles, 2mm in diameter, viewing distance 30 cm) between 1 and 9 were randomly selected and presented for 100 ms in a 4x4 matrix. The task was to press the digit key corresponding to the number of items that were presented as soon as possible. The time of key press from the beginning of the presentation was recorded together with the digit of the key for each of the 170 trials (20 for each item number except item number 1, which was presented only 10 times.) The actual item number was selected randomly.

The result of the test was presented by the instrument by 4 numbers: the basic response time T in seconds for one item, the time per item t in seconds defined by the response time divided by the item number averaged for item numbers 4 to 8, the percentage of correct responses P for item numbers 4 to 8, and the effective recognition speed ERS defined by P/t. (Sometimes we will use simply "effective recognition".)

Altogether, 219 control subjects were recruited from German schools (see Table 1). Poor performance, i. e. grades above 4 on a scale of 1 (best) to 6 in one or more respects was used as a criterion for exclusion. The subjects were classified into 4 age groups as shown in table 1.

Table 1. Development and Deficits: Number of subjects of the 3 groups divided into 4 age groups

Age / years	7 – 8	9 - 10	11 - 13	14 - 17
Control 219	35 (18/17)	36 (20/16)	62 (36/26)	86 (54/32)
Dyslexia 117	10 (6/4)	41 (23/18)	53 (17/36)	13 (8/5)
Dyscalculia 157	21 (14/7)	60 (32/28)	67 (32/35)	9 (8/1)

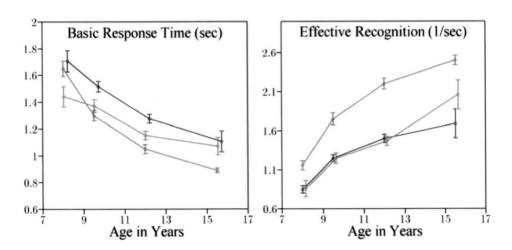

Figure 1. Age curves of the the basic response time (left) and the effective recognition speed (right). The values of the controls are shown in green, those of the dyslexics in red, and those of the children with dyscalculia in blue. Vertical bars indicate the confidence intervals

Using a correlation analysis reveals that from the 4 variables defined above only two are statistically independent. One describes the basic response time T, the other describes the speed of the performance for items between 4 and 8. Here we decided to use ERS, because both variables P and t contribute.

Fig. 1 (teeg-kdl.pcx) shows the age curves of the two independent variables T and ERS. The curves show an improvement of the performance of the task over age. In other words: at the beginning of school at the age of 6 years the capacity of subitizing and number counting is by no means completely developed. The development lasts until adulthood. The development evident from the age curves was confirmed by analysis of variances (ANOVAs) of the variables. This confirms earlier findings on subitizing and counting processes in young children (Svenson and Sjöberg, 1978).

DEFICITS

The same test of subitizing was applied to 117 children with dyslexia and 157 children with dyscalculia (see Table 1). The criterion for being included in one or the other of the two test groups were obtained from the grades in school. In any case all grades had to be within the normal range with the exception of reading, spelling, or math, which were require to fall below the normal range, i.e. at 5 or 6 at a 1 to 6 scale. For a subset of children we had the scores of intelligence tests. These had also to be in the normal range, i. e. above 80.

The age curves of the two groups are also shown in Fig. 1 (teeg-kdl.pcx) for the basic response time (left side) and for the effective recognition speed (right side). Clearly the development of the test children runs behind that of the controls. The discrepancy is evident for the dyscalculia children in both variables and it increases with age. The dyslexic children seem to have only slight deficits concerning the basic response time, while the effective recognition speed exhibits also clear deficits.

Percentage of children performing outside the normal range was found by counting the number of test children whose T-values were above and whose ERS-values were below the 16 percentile of the controls.

The Fig. 2 shows these percentages for the variable T (left side) and for the variable ERS (right side). Note, that by definition this measure implies that 2x16% of the control subjects perform outside the "normal" range and that the 16 percentile corresponds to 1 standard deviation of a normal distribution. The green lines in the figure were obtained from the control subjects and indicate the level of the 16 percentile.

The Fig. 2 confirms the results shown in Fig. 1: both groups contain large percentages of subjects performing outside the normal range. The percentage depends on age and group.

The main difference between the two test groups is obtained in the basic response time: in the dyslexia group only low percentages have problems with responding fast enough. In fact, in the younger groups of dyslexics none of the subjects was outside the normal range. Considering the effective recognition speed the group of children with dyslexia contains also smaller numbers of subjects outside the normal range as compared with the children with dyscalculia.

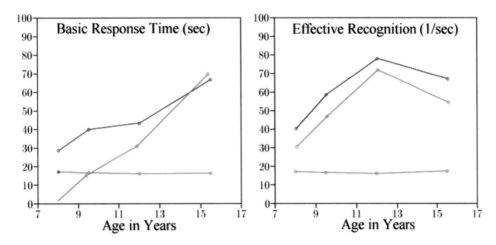

Figure 2. The percentages of children performing outside the normal range are shown as a function of age.

Analysing subitizing separately, by looking at the response times and correctness of responses for item numbers 2, 3, and 4 showed that the children with dyslexia and with dyscalculia exhibit developmental deficits even with the small item numbers.

TRAINING

To overcome the deficits in subitizing the test task was modified and given the children for daily practice at home for a period of 321 weeks including the week ends. Children performing the test task below their age range (below the 16 percentile) were included in the training groups.

The difficulty of the training task was modified by increasing the maximum number of items from 3 in steps up to 9 and by decreasing the presentation time from 300ms at the beginning down to100ms. The training program was implemented in a s mall box such the children could do the training every day for about 10 min at home.

The children had to perform a pre-training session and a post-training session using the original difficulty of the test task. The training devices stored all the data and a training protocol was down-loaded, when the instruments were given back to the laboratory. This enabled to see the course of the training directly day by day and session by session. Pre- and post-training values were analysed.

The Table 2 gives the number of subjects contributing to the corresponding study of children with dyslexia and dyscalculia, respectively. Subjects above age 14 were too small in number, therefore only 3 age groups could be used in the analysis of the pre- and post-training data.

Fig. 3 shows the pre-and post-training curves of the variables T and ERS obtained from the children with dyscalculia. Both, the basis response times and the effective recognition were improved in all age groups.

Comparing the post-training data with those of the control groups of the same age revealed, that about 85% of the subjects reached the normal range, i.e. they reached the 16 percentile or more of the controls. We also analysed subitizing directly by comparing the pre- and post-values for item numbers of 2, 3 and 4, separately. The result was, that this aspect of the test task was also improved in all age groups.

The curves for the dyslexics are very similar and therefore they are not shown here. In fact, it seems that the training affects subitizing and number counting by about the same amount irrespective of whether the subjects had reading or spelling problems or problems with basic arithmetic skills.

Table 2. Training: Number of subjects of the 3 groups divided into 3 age groups

Age / years	7 - 8	9 - 10	11 – 13
Controls 133	35 (18/17)	36 (20/16)	62 (36/26)
Dyslexia 140	45 (17/28)	52 (22/30)	43 (11/32)
Dyscalculia 74	25 (10/15)	30 (17/13)	19 (5/14)

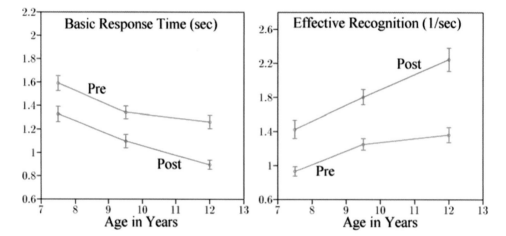

Figure 3. The age curves of the pre-and post-training values of the basic response time (left) and the effective recognition speed (right) of the children with dyscalculia show improvements for all age groups. The vertical bars indicate the confidence intervals.

TRANSFER

The basic arithmetic skills of a group of children with dyscalculia (Gr I) were examined before and after the training. A control group (Gr II) was also examined but during the first period of the study they were not allowed to practice the training-task. After the Gr I had completed the training, the Gr II was given the training also. The children (N = 21) were 7.5 to 9 years old and formed a single age group. (The analysis of any possible age effects showed no significant correlations).

Children with poor performances when operating with small numbers were included. The DEMAT-test consisting of 10 subtests was used for all children before and after their training period. Their other competences, however, were in the normal range of the classes they were visiting at school.

The mathematical competence of both groups was tested before the study (T0), after the first training period (T1), and after the second training period (T2).

Fig. 4 shows on the left side the differences between the score points before and after the first training period of Gr I (the waiting period of Gr II). While the training group exhibits a profit of more than 3 points the waiting Gr II did not show any improvement. The second pair of columns show the differences of points at the end of the second period, whenre Gr II did the training and Gr I visited school without further training.

Now the Gr I gained another 3 points reaching a total profit of about 6 points altogether. These children now improved their mathematical competence by just visiting school.. Such improvement was not obtained by the Gr II during the first period, when they visited school but without a previous training. Gr II due to their training gained also more than 3 points. After another 6 weeks the members of Gr II were again examined. Now they reached a total improvement of about 6 points, about as many as the Gr I.

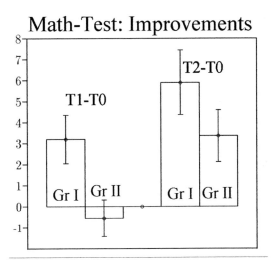

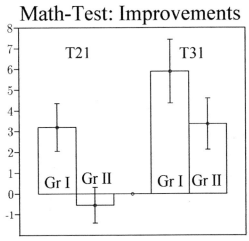

Figure 4. The transfer of the training to basic mathematical competence. The columns show the differences of points scored by the subjects after the first training period (T1-T0) and after the second period (T2-T0).

DISCUSSION

The sequence of studies described in this chapter has shown that a basic visual capacity, subitizing and visual counting by memory, develops until the age of about 18 years. While this finding is not completely new (s. Introduction), we wanted to ensure that the present method shows the development in the age range of 7 to 17 years and we wanted to establish the mean values and their scatter to be able to compare these measures with those obtained from certain groups of children with learning problems.

The investigation of children with specific learning problems (dyslexia or dyscalculia) may suffer from developmental deficits, when tested for subitizing and number counting by memory using the standard test. Not all of these children exhibit the deficit and not all of them have the same amount of deficit. The percentages of affected children varies from 30 to 80% depending on age and group.

When given a training of subitizing for 3 weeks about 85% of the subjects were able to improve their capacity and reached the range of an age matched control group. The training transfers to improvements of basic mathematical skills.

While this study was conducted without a placebo group some of the effects may be due to the fact, that the test children experienced the fact that they were successful with the training itself and transferred this experience to their mathematical skills. However, the detailed analysis of the subtests of the DEMAT shows, that not all subtest yielded improvements suggesting that only those subfunctions of the test were affected which rely on subitizing and a sense of number.

Moreover, this study was intended to see whether the methods of diagnosis and training could be successfully applied in everyday school. It does not necessarily contribute to a theoretical understanding the phenomenon of dyslexia or dyscalculia. Yet, the results support the view, that such a basic cognitive skill makes an important contribution to learn simple operations with numbers.

Earlier studies on the role of saccade control on reading and of auditory deficits on spelling have yielded similar results. It seems that processing of auditory, visual and optomotor information in the brain improves during the total developmental period until adulthood. Deficits in one or more of these domains contribute to learning problems, which are reduced when the deficits are treated by daily practice.

REFERENCES

Balakrishnan, J. D. and Ashby, F. G. (1991). Is subitizing a unique numerical ability? *Perception and Psychophysics* 50, 555-564.

Biscaldi, M., Fischer, B., and Hartnegg, K. (2000). Voluntary saccade control in dyslexia. *Perception,* 29, 509-521.

Cowan, N. (2001). The magical number 4 in short-term memory: A reconsideration of mental storage capacity. *Behav.Brain Sci.* 26, 87-116.

Dehaene, S. (1999). *Der Zahlensinn*. Basel: Birkhäuser Verlag.

Fischer, B. and Hartnegg, K. (2004). On the development of low level auditory discrimination and deficits in dyslexia. *Dyslexia* 10[2], 105-118.

Fischer, B. and Hartnegg, K. (2000). Effects of visual training on saccade control in dyslexia. *Perception* 29, 531-542.

Fischer, B., Hartnegg, K., and Mokler, A. (2000). Dynamic visual perception of dyslexic children. *Perception* 29, 523-530.

Jensen, E. M., Reese, E. P., and Reese, T. W. (1950). The subitizing and counting of visually presented fields of dots. *Journal of Psychology: Interdisciplinary and Applied* 30, 363-392.

Mandler, G. and Shebo, B. J. (1982). Subitizing: An analysis of its component processes. *J.Exp.Psychol.Gen.* 11, 1-22.

Schäffler, T., Sonntag, J., and Fischer, B. (2004). The effect of daily practice on low level auditory discrimination, phonological skills, and spelling in dyslexia. *Dyslexia* 10[2], 119-130.

Silverman, I. W. and Rose, A. P. (1980). Subitizing and counting skills in 3-year-olds. *Developmental Psychology* 16, 539-540.

Stanescu-Cosson, R., Pinel, P., van de Moortele, P. F., Le Bihan, D., Cohen, L., and Dehaene, S. (2000). Understanding dissociation in dyscalculia: a brain imaging study of the impact of number size on the cerebral network for exact and approximate calculation. *Brain* 123, 2240-2255.

Starkey, P. and Cooper, R. G. (1995). The development of subitizing in young children. *British J. Developmental Psychology* 13, 399-420.

Starkey, P. and Cooper, R. G. (1980). Perception of number by human infants. *Science* 210, 1033-1035.

Svenson, O. and Sjöberg, K. (1978). Subitizing and counting processes in young children. *Scand. J. Psychol.* 19, 247-250.

Trick, L. M., Enns, J. T., and Brodeur, D. a. (1996). Life span changes in visual enumeration: The number discrimination task. *Developmental Psychology* 35[5], 925-932.

Trick, L. M. and Phylyshyn, Z. W. (1994). Why are small and large numbers enumerated differently? A limited-capacity preattentive stage in vision. *Psychol.Rev.* 101, 80-102.

In: Dyslexia in Children: New Research
Editor: Christopher B. Hayes, pp. 103-122

ISBN 1-59454-969-9
© 2006 Nova Science Publishers, Inc.

Chapter 6

CURRENT DYSLEXIA RESEARCH SEEN IN THE LIGHT OF IMRE LAKATOS' PHILOSOPHY OF RESEARCH PROGRAMMES

Turid Helland[1] and Kjetil Rommetveit[2]

[1] Faculty of Psychology
Center for the Study of the Sciences and the Humanities
[2] University of Bergen

ABSTRACT

In this paper different fields of dyslexia research will be analysed in the view of Lakatos "research programmes". The aim is two-folded; to try and see if his intended meaning of "research programmes" is applicable to dyslexia research; and to use his philosophy of science to gain a meta-view, and hence better insight into the current status of dyslexia research. The high frequency of dyslexia in the population, its educational implications, and its many intertwining scientific and clinical aspects, invite for a useful framework to organise the knowledge.

INTRODUCTION

In this paper different research approaches to dyslexia will tentatively be analysed according to Imre Lakatos' (1922-1974) philosophy of research programmes. Dyslexia is a multifaceted disorder involving several fields of research and clinical approaches, which are more or less in communication with each other. It was first described at the turn of the 19th century as a case of word-blindness, or strephosymbolia, by the British medical doctor Morgan (Morgan 1892), and has since then emerged much research. Reading and writing are cultural activities of modern society and hence cannot be said to be a human brain activity refined by evolution. On the other hand, there is a general agreement that reading and writing impairment, dyslexia, is a language based disorder, and thus related to language activities in the brain.

Since Morgan's description, several professional fields have become involved in the search for a better understanding of this impairment, this including educators, sociologists, psychologists, and biologists. "Paradoxes in behaviour give clues to the underlying causes of the behaviour. That is why dyslexia is one of the key disorders in the systematic investigation of the architecture of the mind and its basis in the brain" (Frith 1999), p. 4). This phrase points to the uniqueness of dyslexia as a specific impairment within cognitive functioning, invisible and unobservable except for during reading and writing activities, but highly socially invalidating. This is perhaps one of the main reasons why so many different fields have been engaged in dyslexia research and intervention. As a result several fields have evolved research based on their own scientific "paradigms", with various effort and outcomes of co-operation and common understanding.

In this paper different fields of dyslexia research will be analysed in the view of Lakatos "research programmes". The aim is two-folded; to try and see if his intended meaning of "research programmes" is applicable to dyslexia research; and to use his philosophy of science to gain a meta-view, and hence better insight into the current status of dyslexia research. The high frequency of dyslexia in the population, its educational implications, and its many intertwining scientific and clinical aspects, invite for a useful framework to organise the knowledge.

LAKATOS' PHILOSOPHY OF SCIENCE

Lakatos developed his theories of research programmes as an attempt to improve on, and overcome, the objections to Popper's and Kuhn's theories of science. According to Lakatos, Popperian falsificationism had failed to place hypotheses within their proper historical context, and Kuhn's paradigms was "mob psychology", undermining progress and the rules by which science is conducted (Lakatos 1970), pp. 91-195)

The philosophy of Lakatos was distinctive for its period: together with Popper and Kuhn he sought out alternative explanations of scientific rationality to the long prevailing account given by logical positivism. Along with Kuhn, Lakatos acknowledged the central role of historiography to the philosophy of science. The logical positivists, but also Popper, had sought out rigorous and a-historical standards of rationality that may have gone well with logic, but which nevertheless gave poor descriptions of the ways in which scientific research was actually carried out. But being as he was deeply influenced by Popper's rationalism, Lakatos could not accept the relativistic and non-normative conclusions that seemed to follow from Kuhn's main work, The Structure of Scientific Revolutions (Kuhn 1970). The philosophy of research programs, therefore, was Lakatos' attempt at situating Popperian norms of scientific research within historically situated practices of research. Due to the fundamental historical character of investigation, the question was not so much the classical 'what is science'? It was rather 'what accounts for scientific progress and the growth of knowledge?' In what follows, we give a short description of the main criteria that the theory of research programs laid down in order to answer this question (Lakatos, 1970).

The hard core of a programme consists of basic theoretical principles that are not to be questioned if the research is to get going in the first place. It cannot be falsified in the way proposed by Popper. Hence, the hard core is not directly applied in the research, but it is the presupposition of this research. An example of a hard core of a scientific program may be the central role ascribed to DNA in inheritance and the development of new cells in the organism. As knowledge grows, the hard core may expand and develop. It may not, however, change it's principles in a substantial way. In that case, we cannot any longer talk about the same programme.

The hard core is put into practice through the programme's *protective belt.* By this concept, Lakatos means the concrete theories and hypotheses to be tested by the actual research. The protective belt is also to be regarded as supplied by theories from related fields, by the available technological and instrumental means, by auxiliary hypotheses and mathematical theories. This part of the program may, in contradistinction to the hard core, be changed and revised continuously as the research goes along. It may not, however, violate the principles of the hard core.

The protective belt is carried out through the programme's *positive heuristic,* which suggests plans and concrete methods for carrying out the research as well as establishing methodological strategies and hypothesis for the research. The *negative heuristic* states that the basic, hard core must not be rejected or modified.

Scientific methodology must be discussed from two points of view: the work done *within* a single research programme, and the comparison *between* competing research programmes. This involves that the expansion and modification of its protective belt is permissible as long as it is not *ad hoc*, and as long as it does not violate the hard core of the program. An ad hoc modification means that the theory cannot be tested in any way that is not also a test of the original theory. The modified theory is not ad hoc when it leads to new tests, i.e. it can be tested independently. Modifications or additions to the protective belt of a research programme must be independently testable, by fresh tests and hence the possibility of new discoveries.

Hence, according to Lakatos two kinds of hypotheses are ruled out: ad hoc hypotheses and hypotheses that violate the hard core. The fact that any part of a complex theory might be responsible for an apparent falsification, poses a serious problem for the Popperian falsificationist, as the inability to locate the source of the trouble may result in unmethodological chaos. Lakatos' account of science is adequately structured to avoid that consequence. Order is maintained by the stability of the hard core of a programme and by the positive heuristic that accompanies it.

The comparison between research programmes is more problematic than within a research programme, since the degree of success within a research programme is to be evaluated by its progress or lack of progress. The time factor represents a major difficulty in this respect: how much time must pass before it can be decided that a programme has degenerated, that it is incapable of leading to the discovery of new phenomena? It is always possible that some ingenious modification of its protective belt will lead to some spectacular discovery that will revitalise the programme. Because scientific growth of knowledge is ultimately a question of historically situated processes of learning, one can never make the unqualified claim that one research programme is "better" than a rival. Still, the relative merits of the programmes can be decided retrospectively: "Methodology is wedded to history…since methodology is nothing but a rational reconstruction of history, of the growth of knowledge" (Lakatos 1970,1978). See also Chamers (1982)), for a further discussion.

Critical comments. The criteria of Lakatos are recognisable in scientific publications of clinical and experimental work. To be submitted, a research paper has to have an introduction, showing the theoretic and empirical base of the new study. This should compare to the hard core, the negative heuristic and the protective belt within the actual field of research. The hypotheses set forth, the method and result parts, with the summarising discussion, should cover the last criteria of a research programme, the positive heuristic and the method part. At a larger scale, the hard core, the negative heuristic, and the protective belt seem to define the research programme, while the positive heuristic and the methodology seem to define the vitality and the progress of the programme. This comparison immediately raises the question of what extension a programme should have to fulfil the criteria of a research programme set by Lakatos. In his description of research programmes that do not fulfil his criteria, Freudianism and Marxism are held out, which at least gives an indication of how Lakatos himself dimensioned a research programme (Chamers 1982).

Paul Feyerabend criticised Lakatos for having failed to offer a clear-cut criterion for the rejection of any coherent research programme, or for choosing between rival research programmes (Feyerabend 1975). He described Lakatos' methodology as "a verbal ornament, as a memorial to happier times when it was still thought possible to run a complex and often catastrophic business like science by following a few simple and 'rational' rules" (Chamers 1982). For instance, Feyerabend will be liable to ascribe a much more central and positive function to ad hoc hypothisation than is Lakatos (Feyerabend, 1975, pp.14-15). In the following an effort will be made to sort out different programmes within dyslexia research according to Lakatos' criteria. If this is clarifying and rendering truth to current dyslexia research, credit will be given to Lakatos' efforts at structuring research. Conversely, if his criteria goes unwarranted, credit will be given to Feyerabend's criticism.

DYSLEXIA

Dyslexia is described as a word-decoding impairment and a temporal processing deficit. It is also described as a multifaceted disorder. The term suffers from a variety of definitions reflecting the various professional viewpoints involved in dyslexia research.

Clinically dyslexia cannot be observed other than by reading and writing behaviour. Like other clinical impairments a wide variety of different underlying impairments may cause dyslexia. This is illustrated in Figure 1.

Knivsberg (1997) describes the figure in this way: "The figure illustrates three basic causal models. The first one, on the left hand side, shows one biological factor (O) that gives rise to two cognitive dysfunctions (C1, C2), and these dysfunctions lead to two behavioural abnormalities (S1, S2). This model resembles the letter A, and is referred to as an A-type causal model. The second is an X-type model, indicating that two biological factors (O1, O2) may effect just one cognitive dysfunction, C, but this dysfunction may lead to two abnormalities at the behavioural level (S1, S2). The third model, the V-type, indicates that two biological factors (O1, O2) may result in two cognitive dysfunctions (C1, C2), and these may have the same effect on the behaviour thus leading to one abnormal trait (S)" (p.15).

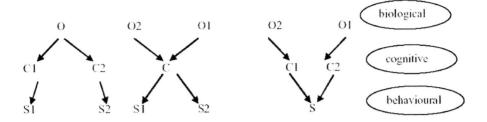

Figure 1. Basic casual models for developmental psychopathology. From (Morton and Frith 1995)

Dyslexia is mainly diagnosed by educational specialists by assessment of functional reading and writing (collecting behavioural data, level S), data from cognitive testing (collecting data for inferring cognitive assets and deficits, level C), and collected qualitative data of birth and pre-natal status, heredity (level O), language development, school history, parental and school support (teachers, classmates, special educational support), teaching strategies and the child's self esteem (collecting environmental data). Also, but still quite rare, neuro-psychological testing (C), and brain scanning (O) is used, mainly to exclude the possibility of brain damage. Dyslexia should not be diagnosed from any one of these areas alone. However, as this shows, the tester should be familiar with fields involving biological, neurological, cognitive, behavioural, sociological and cultural factors relevant to dyslexia assessment and intervention.

As pointed out by (Frith 1997) and (Lundberg, Tønnesen and Austad 1999), several current fields of cognitive research involve different "levels of explanation". They both hold that links between biological, cognitive and behavioural levels are needed for a better understanding of dyslexia. This interaction is shown in Figure 2.

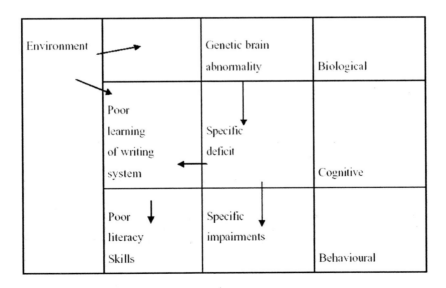

Figure 2. Basic causal modelling diagram. From (Frith 1997).

Behaviour can be explained by cognitive dysfunctions, and cognitive dysfunctions can be explained by brain dysfunctions. However, this linkage has to be evaluated within the context of environmental and cultural influences of the dyslexic individual.

Four Different Approaches to Dyslexia Research in the Perspective of Lakatos' Philosophy of Science

In this section four different fields of dyslexia research will be described. The word "field" is used, because it is uncertain that they are research programmes in Lakatos' sense. The three first fields are in accordance with the three levels shown in Figure 1. Frith (ibid) also includes "environment" as a fourth field, not at a separate level, but as a field involving all the other three levels. In the present paper the "environmental" level will be represented by the sociological approach to dyslexia. As the reader will see, each of the fields is described by the plural as "approaches". This underlines an important factor, namely that within each field there are several sub-fields, or approaches. This again is troublesome as to the question raised earlier, of the extensiveness, or inclusiveness, of a programme. For the sake of clarification, and to adjust to Lakatos' structure, the descriptions given here of each field are simplified, with little or no attention given to cross-over approaches. Thus, the qualified reader within dyslexia research will find the overview incomplete, but – hopefully – with some basic truth in it.

BIOLOGICAL/MEDICAL APPROACHES

Hard Core

Biological approaches study theories on structures and functions of the brain. As to dyslexia, a brain researcher or geneticist will naturally ask the question if structural, functional or developmental deficits are related to the language areas of the brain. This hard core of biological approaches to dyslexia is then carried out in research on brain structures, functions and development, and on genetics and heredity.

Usually biological research programmes are not devoted to dyslexia alone, but to a diversity of clinical conditions. At least studies of brain development and genetics in dyslexia seem to be part of more widespread studies on several impaired groups. Thus the dyslexia research is part of a larger programme. An example of this is the large scale studies conducted by Geschwindt, Behan and Galaburda on the effects of auto-immune disorders on brain development (Behan and Geschwind 1985; Geschwind and Galaburda 1985). As to studies on heredity, the picture is somewhat different. The large twin study conducted by Olson and his collegues at the University of Colorado, is an example of a research programme devoted to dyslexia only (Olson 1999).

Negative Heuristic

The negative heuristic should then be that dyslexia is one among several disabilities of a constitutional origin caused either by heredity (genes) or brain dysfunction. In this sense research is focused more on causality than on intervention. Causality is inferred from possible brain deviancies. Thus the main part of this research must be labelled basal research.

Protective Belt

Imaging studies, genetic studies, or studies of the brain linked to pre-natal status or premature birth are closely linked to medical studies and professions. Thus the medical profession is a prerequisite for this type of research, which to a larger degree than in the other fields helps to define the protective belt. However, as will be discussed later, for several studies this is not necessarily the case. There are very often multi-professional groups behind many of these studies.

Positive Heuristics

Similar dysfunctions may be caused by a magnitude of different underlying neurological deficits, the aetiology of which need to be clarified to implement the right remedial programmes. Therefore it is essential to clarify assets and deficits in the structure of the actual brain. Historically, research within this area gained useful insight through neurological research on aphasia and other acquired brain dysfunctions. Today one will be careful not to draw conclusions from acquired dysfunctions to developmental dysfunctions. According to Frith brain researchers and geneticists are rapidly accumulating new knowledge and mappings for further research (Frith 1997). Examples are the Galaburda, Behan, Geschwindt (GBG) hypotheses on abnormal structures of the planum temporale (Geschwind 1979; Behan and Geschwind 1985; Galaburda 1990), the identification of cellular migration abnormalities (Livingstone, Rosen, Drislane and Galaburda 1991), the genetic linkage studies with dyslexic families having identified regions in chromosomes 15, 1 and 6 (Fagerheim, Tønnesen, Raemaekers and Lubs 1999), and through the quickly progressing imaging studies with PET, fMRI or MEG scanning of the brain. Another biological field, gaining renewed interest, concerns the effect of otitis media with effusion (OME), on language development, and its prevalence in dyslexic children. Also, intervention studies conducted by brain researchers have shown effects of intensive training of auditory processing in the planum temporale by sound and letter exercises (Tallal 2000).

Methodology within a Research Programme

Most studies within the biological domain are experimental on relatively small samples. As a criterion for inclusion, or exclusion, the dyslexia definition by the World Federation of Neurology (WFN) of 1968 is applied, which among other things claims that the subjects should be within normal I. Q.- range. For the sake of research simplicity and comparability, often only right-handed boys are included (see i.e. (Paulesu, Démonet, Fazio et al. 2001). Objective task dependent tests are being applied. The studies are published as articles in international journals, thus being subjected to strict critical remarks by its reviewers. It is expected that the introduction part of the study gives the theoretical basis through reporting to other accepted studies. This is an assurance against what Lakatos calls ad hoc hypothisation. The methodological parts of the studies are expected to be described in detail and by certain conventions, to ensure that the study can be replicated. This should secure the claim of being independent testable.

Within brain imaging, new barriers are rapidly broken, not at least by advances in brain computer technology. As to genetics, the race for breaking the genetic code is also echoed in dyslexia research. However, within these and other high cost projects, research is also quickly published through the Internet, which can be a threat to the quality insurance of the journals. This may violate either the two demands of Lakatos, of ad hoc, or of violation to the hard core, by its rapid and unreviewed publications. Or, even more radically; the pace and the complexity of developments within these fields of research may be seen as transgressing the boundaries of a Lakatosian reconstruction. From the point of view of research programmes then, these developments may be evaluated negatively, as breaking the basic norms of scientific research. Alternatively, they may be seen as confirming Feyerabend's criticism of Lakatos: there is no single fact of the matter as to what qualifies as good science.

Comparison of Research Programmes

Within the biological field the refinement of brain mapping technology and the genetic programmes seem to be vigorously expanding, while the research legacy of i.e. the GBG-hypotheses of auto-immune disorders, seems to be less vigorous. However, a growing interest in the role of the right hemisphere and the development of pre-mature babies, may give a raise to research on environmental influences in foetus. But as a conclusion: brain mapping and genetics are spectacular and prestigious (and high cost research), in this sense giving a lead over other areas of dyslexia research at the moment. As remarked, high degrees of uncertainty are involved in attempts at evaluating these developments.

COGNITIVE APPROACHES

Hard Core

According to (Frith 1997) there is a big gap between an individual child's behaviour and the methods of instruction it has been subjected to. This gap is what cognitive psychology has claimed as its own. Especially cognitive neuroscience is promising in that the cognitive level will connect known behavioural signs to biological and environmental factors that have an influence on development. This means that theories of learning, attention, memory, executive functions, intelligence and language are essential in cognitive theories, with basis in normal cognitive processing. A good theory will link the cognitive processes to brain processes and environmental influences.

Since dyslexia is viewed as a linguistically based impairment with weak phonological awareness as the core problem (Vellutino 1991; The Orton Dyslexia Society 1994), much research the last 10-20 years has focused on the different aspects of phonology in dyslexic subjects of different age groups and backgrounds. An overweight of the research and attention has been focused on reading over writing. The interaction with the environment is crucial as to what effect the impairment may have on the individual. Therefore, the effects of early intervention programs have been given much focus, and also longitudinal studies to find how the core deficit exposes itself at different ages. Studies of comorbidity with other cognitive deficits are accepted within the cognitive approach.

Negative Heuristic

As to dyslexia, one will naturally ask the question if functional cognitive deficits in any of the above mentioned areas are more closely linked to dyslexia than any of the other. Frith also points to two opposite approaches that are taken by different theoreticians: either to identify the specific component responsible for the specific test failure, or to doubt there is a specific problem and to look for a more general problem. Frith points to an abundance of research supporting the phonological deficit hypothesis as causal modelling of dyslexia. She says that there is an overweight of scientific evidence for this hypothesis as of a specific, persistent and universal deficit (Frith 1985). During the last 20 years this has been accepted as a core problem, and is also given definitional status. However, a main principle within this field is that dyslexic impairment is inferred from the results of cognitive tasks that are regarded crucial to dyslexia. Within this field research seems to be equally divided between basal and applied research.

Protective Belt

The phonological deficits are assessed by a diversity of cognitive tasks, involving phonological processing. These may be rapid automatic naming, verbal learning and memory, non-word repetition, phoneme awareness, or object naming. There is little controversy in that deficits in any of these areas are closely, and perhaps causally, linked to biological or environmental factors, as shown in Figure 2.

Positive Heuristic

Unlike the biological field, research within these areas is more often focused on dyslexia alone, and not on a diversity of clinical conditions. Efforts are being made to sort out tests that assess more clearly each of the areas, directed towards the specificity of dyslexia. Recently also the sway of the pendulum seems to open up for other causal hypotheses of dyslexia within the cognitive approach. One can see renewed acceptance for a possible visual deficit hypothesis, and also a cerebellar abnormality hypothesis, pointing to poor motor control of eye and hand movements crucial to reading and writing performance (Stein and Walsh 1997; Nicolson and Fawcett 1999; Stein 2000; Beaton 2004). In addition to this there is an ongoing research on comorbidity with other cognitive deficits, as SLI or dyscalculia (Helland and Asbjornsen 2003, 2004), and in disconnecting dyslexia from the discrepancy criteria of IQ and reading and writing performance (Siegel 1992; Fletcher, Shaywitz, Shankweiler et al. 1994). This opens up for research on other populations with a possible dyslexic condition.

Methodology within a Research Programme

Also within the cognitive domain a large portion of the research is experimental and on small samples. However, some principal differences to the biological methodology are often seen. The samples may be clinical, adjusted to a definition that does not necessarily exclude as strictly by the I.Q.-level as the WFN-definition. This goes for the definition by the (The British Dyslexia Association 1998). Standardised tests are being applied. Also, studies applying a qualitative approach are seen. The studies are published as articles in international journals of cognition, and thus being subjected to critical reviews. It is expected that at least the introduction part of the study gives the theoretical basis through reporting to other accepted studies. This is an assurance against what Lakatos calls the formation of ad hoc hypotheses. As to the method part of the study, this should be reported in detail, so that the study can be replicated. This should secure the claim of being independently testable. Since this research is not high cost, spectacular or competitive in the same way as within the biological research, the Internet publications do not appear to the same extent.

The Comparison of Research Programmes

The cognitive field within dyslexia research is today by far the most dominant, in the sense that its identification of what dyslexia is, is widely accepted and applied as research definition by the other fields. However, so much work is done on the phonological part that there may be signs of exhaustion. The future prospect of this field lies in its own willingness to accept other cognitive aspects of dyslexia than the linguistic/phonological one. Also, development of phonological tasks for functional imaging studies, and for tapping what is specific for different languages (transparent/opaque, syntagmatic/paradigmatic, analytic/synthetic) seem to be prosperous. Critical remarks are that by sampling dyslexics through phonological impairment, one will always find some linguistic impairment (Tønnessen 1995, 1997). Also, there may be a controversy in what linguists define as "phonological" and the somewhat wider definition used by other professionals, including i.e. morphology and syllables as phonological elements (Uppstad 2005). These critical remarks need to be taken seriously and sorted out.

BEHAVIOURAL APPROACHES

Hard Core

The behavioural approaches are founded on analyses and categorisations of functional reading and writing performance. In contrast to the cognitive approach, equally much emphasis is put on reading and writing performance.

Research Programmes

Within this approach, the reading and writing performances are categorised according to types of mistakes, as dysphonetic, dyseidic or mixed (Boder 1969, 1973), as auditory, visual or audio-visual, or according to relative strength (Gjessing 1977, 1986), as P-type (perceptually strong) or L-type (linguistically strong) (Bakker 1992), or by process analyses in comparison to stages on a model of normal acquisition of reading and writing (i.e. the dual route model). The three first systems of classification were dominant both in research and in clinical work until the late 70s, when the phonological approach gradually became dominant. The process analytic model of the dual route is closely connected to the phonological approach, but with analyses of functional reading processes as its diagnostic tool. Typical of these approaches is that they are closely linked to the names and personal impact of their "founders". They also have pedagogical books of instruction and programmes of interventions attached to their assessment tasks.

Negative Heuristic

The basic assumption is that dyslexia is a deficit manifested through reading and writing performances. Within the sets of classification the deficits are not only related to modalities, but also to pedagogical instruction and to emotional status. This has to be clarified through interviews with the subject, parents and teachers. The research within this field is fundamentally applied research, due to its offspring from and closeness to educators and the school system.

Protective Belt

An important part of these approaches is the closeness to practical work with the dyslexic pupil within the educational system. The classifications are deeply manifested in many teachers' understanding of dyslexia, at least in the western world. In some research positive correlation between the auditory and visual sub-grouping and respective modality weakness is found. However, during the last 20 years any visual deficit hypothesis has been denied, as several studies have not found any correlates (Vellutino 1978, 1979, 1991). Thus the hard core of the modality related approaches has been refuted by a dominant part of dyslexia researchers, which means degeneration of research progress, according to Lakatos. The processing approach, however, with its close connection to the phonological research, has prospered with the progression made by this field of research.

Positive Heuristic

In contrast to the biological and cognitive fields, cognitive deficits are inferred through reading and writing behaviour. For example, phonetically incorrect spelling may be a sign of auditory/dysphonetic impairment, while phonetically correct, but orthographically incorrect spelling, may indicate a visual/dyseidic deficit. There is little disagreement on the auditory significance in dyslexia. However, and not at least, the disregard of a visual deficit component in dyslexia has been objected to among language teachers, finding specific spelling mistakes in verbally and reading competent pupils inexplicable by a deficit in the phonological system. Examples of these objections are "caught" spelled as /kaut/, "what" as /wat/, "laugh" as /laf/. Thus the renewed interest in visual factors in dyslexia, as mentioned in the biological and cognitive parts, may lead to a revival of the visual subgroup in dyslexia. Differences in occipital, and hence visual activation, is seen in brain imaging when comparing dyslexic subjects to controls. Thus Lakatos' argument, that even if a set of theories and core assumptions has been falsified it is worth while keeping, as long as it offers useful predictions (Chamers 1982), is encouraging for the clinician/pedagocical opponents of the phonological deficits hypothesis.

Although the phonological deficit hypothesis is seen across languages, there are studies showing that different languages affect functional reading and writing in different ways (Wimmer 1993; Goswami 1999; Landerl 2003; Hagtvet, Helland and Lyster 2005). Also, most research is done on mono-linguals for the sake of validity. A growing interest is seen in multi-lingualism, and dialectal influences (Peer and Reid 2000; Helland and Kaasa 2005). There is also an initial discussion on the definition of "phonology", where the different professions define the term differently (Uppstad 2005).

Methodology within a Research Programme

Compared to the biological and cognitive approaches, this field is characterised by being applied rather than experimental. This is not surprising, since this approach has its offspring in, and has remained closer to, the clinical and educational fields than the other two approaches. Its classification system based on reading and writing performance is still deeply rooted in educational thinking. The auditory deficit hypothesis has been strengthened through much biological and cognitive research, while the visual correlates have been difficult to find. This has also been the main arguments against these systems of classification. In this sense research within the auditory/visual dichotomy has been ad hoc. However, some intervention programmes based on the hard core, seem to have been successful. At least this seems to be the case with Bakker's L- and P-type dyslexia, where the intervention programmes are based on the subgrouping from functional performance in reading and writing, combined with cognitive tests, i.e. dichotic listening (Bakker 1992). In addition, follow-up studies have shown significant effects of the intervention programmes, which are constructed from knowledge on cognitive assets and deficits. Also follow-up studies from process-oriented intervention are reporting positive effects.

The Comparison of Research Programmes

Clearly parts of the "functional analyses" programmes seem to have fallen behind, while the "process-analytic" methods have been progressing. However, the time factor is essential in Lakatos' research programmes. The view that there is a need to focus more on other factors than the phonological, along with the rapidly advancing brain imaging technology, may revive research on the visual factor in reading and writing. Also, it is intuitive that both visual and auditory modalities are essential to reading and writing.

In all, the relative strength of these approaches is not in the scientific merits, but in the position it has earned through educational applicability.

SOCIOLOGICAL APPROACHES

Hard Core

According to the sociological approach, there are two incompatible traditional positions on dyslexia, namely the positivistic, diagnostic position, held by the three previously described approaches, and a humanistic position, or "orientation towards normalisation", based on sociological thinking, according to the Norwegian sociologist Per Solvang (Solvang 1995, 1998; 1999). These positions seem to be mutually provocative. The sociological/normalisation approach views dyslexia as an area of knowledge, which is defined by certain interests and agents. The two approaches are shown in Figure 3.

	Principles of causality	Definition of the problem	Problem solving
Diagnostic tradition	Biological	Decoding abilities	Problem oriented and individually adjusted teaching
Tradition of normality	Social	Learning possibilities	Teaching oriented towards mastering, social change

Figure 3. Two traditional approaches to the understanding of reading- and writing impairment (Solvang, 1998).

Negative Heuristic

The normalisation approach has offered two slightly different perspectives on dyslexia (and other medical conditions and handicaps). The first one is a "perspective of crisis", which holds that the experts' diagnoses and interventions undermine the individual's own problem solving abilities and self esteem. Dyslexia as an impairment within the individual does not exist, but is induced upon the child through society, either by incompetent teaching, or the society's demand for diagnoses. According to sociological "labelling theory", the diagnosis represents a conspiracy of interests not primarily to the benefit of the dyslexic individual, but to satisfy the different interests of the actors on the arena; the scientists, the parents, the school system and the judicial system. Consequently, dyslexia as a concept has become a social construct, based on theories of professionalism and power. For instance, as medical doctors "own" the knowledge of medicine, special educators have in their own interest to rule, control and define special educational needs, diagnosis and intervention. The schools and the special needs programmes are viewed as socially biased systems keeping certain social groups in subordinate social positions, excluding them from work and living an autonomous life. By this approach, the society's need for diagnosis will cause the label "dyslexia". The approach is well known in many countries, but only Germany has accepted this view as an "official" viewpoint on dyslexia, after a heated debate in the 1970s.

The second perspective is called a "perspective of negotiation". It is based on sociological studies of areas within traditional medicine. The main idea is that diagnosis and intervention are not dictated by the expert alone, but in an interaction with all the participants on the arena, where all actors view the situation in their own way and act accordingly. This view accepts the existence of dyslexia, but not necessarily as a result of an individual impairment, but just as well as society's failure to meet the child's needs to learn in its interaction with the environment. Learning to read and write are parts of our complex cultural activities, which have to be taken seriously in the way schools conduct the learning processes of the pupils.

Protective Belt

The protective belt is that dyslexia is more or less a construct that should be explained in sociological terms, meaning that it is an artefact kept alive in the interests of involved professionals. The maintenance of the diagnosis is a result of a game theory, where all actors profit, but from their own interests. As a consequence, a constructionistic view on knowledge (cp. Kuhn's paradigms) the diagnosis "dyslexia" is explainable by the needs of the professionals, and thus the concept is mainly a construct. Evidence for this is the increasing number of dyslexics in the educational system, demanding special education, special aids and special adjustments. One argument for this view is that modern computer technology has advanced to give considerable support to reading and writing disabled, which should contribute to a decrease in demand for special educational programmes.

Positive Heuristic

According to Solvang (1999) the international dyslexia research in the humanistic tradition is weak. One of its central persons, Frank Smith, has not published anything in the period 1985-1997, leading to a categorical bias typical of the controversy of the field. Smith is very critical to talking about learning difficulties at all. The pupils can not be defined as problems, but as an important part of the development of the schools. This makes it difficult to criticise the normalising educators by referring to international publications on "reading difficulties". In particular the humanistic approach is weak in Norway, which can not be explained by a limited scientific production alone. It can be explained by social relations, meaning a close interaction between a tradition of special education, official interests and scientific institutions in a small country.

Solvang points to the necessity of strengthening the normalisation perspective, because different approaches to a field of knowledge are in itself stimulating and accumulates knowledge. Then he also points to an important field of dyslexia research with a sociological approach, namely the relationship between special education and jurisdiction. Another important field of sociological research should be how new laws of certifications within manual work affect adult dyslexic employees. Still another field of sociological research should be the dyslexic person in the computerised world; falling behind, or profiting?

Methodology within a Research Programme

According to Lakatos any move is permissible, as long as it does not violate the hard core and is not ad hoc. Solvang's own research on different outcomes of the debate between diagnostic and normalisation approach in Denmark, Sweden and Norway, based on traditional sociological methodology on medicine, seem to satisfy these criteria. However, as Solvang himself points to, much of the argumentation from this point of view has been looked upon as "underdog" in Norway, due to the lack of formal positions among the discussants. But Solvang also sees individuals within the established institutions who in their research take both positions.

Moreover, and as Solvang will know, there have been quite a few studies on the living situation of dyslexics in Scandinavia. These studies are often master theses, based on surveys on large samples (i.e. questionnaires handed out through dyslexia organisations). Being master theses they are rarely published in international journals. By nature, the research within the sociological tradition on dyslexia is applied research.

The Comparison of Research Programmes

From the way the "diagnostic" and the "normalising" traditions are put forth by sociology, the research programs seem to be quite incompatible. However, by looking back at the way Frith gave an overview of dyslexia research (see Figure 1), the environmental approach is given a large and central role in all three "diagnostic" fields. Reading and writing as cultural activities depending on environmental factors seem to comprise a basis in her understanding of the problem of dyslexia. In this context sociology is the expert field on social interaction. However, the dichotomization put forward by the sociological tradition, is not verbalised in the "diagnostic" tradition, and may very well be looked upon as an example of constructionism from these approaches. In other words, a common arena for communication and comparison of research programmes does not seem to exist. But they both mirror ongoing debates, especially among educators.

DISCUSSION

The aim of this meta-study was two-folded; first to see if Lakatos' intended meaning of "research programmes" was applicable to dyslexia research; secondly to apply his philosophy of science to gain a meta-perspective of the field of current dyslexia research.

To see if intended meaning of "research programmes" was applicable to dyslexia research, and in accordance with well-known researchers on dyslexia, the field was divided into four research fields, the biological, the cognitive, the behavioural, and the sociological. The fact that each field is comprised of a variety of different sub-fields had to be overlooked, but is an obvious problem as to how define a research programme.

An effort was made to analyse to what degree each field fulfilled the conditions set by Lakatos to be a research programme. This is tentatively, and as a first trial, summarised in Table 1 below.

Table 1. The degree to which degree each field can be defined as a research program, according to Lakatos

	Hard core	Negative heuristic	Protective belt	Positive heuristic	Methodology	Comp. within	Comp. between
Biol.	+	+	+	+	+	+	+
Cogn.	+	+	+	+	+	+	+
Behav.	+	+	+	–	–	–	–
Sociol.	+	+	+	–	–	–	–

+ (plus) = an overweigh within Lakatos demands; – (minus) = an overweigh not to his demands.

Obviously a model like this lacks important nuances. Nevertheless, some traits become more profiled. All fields seem to suffice as to the hard core, the negative heuristic, and the protective belt. As mentioned earlier, these conditions identify the actual field, or research programme. In this respect all seem to succeed in meeting the demanded criteria. However, only the biological and cognitive fields seem to prosper. The behavioural and the sociological fields seem to fall behind as to expansion. This is not necessarily identical with future failure, since the question of time is important in Lakatos' terminology. The closeness to education in the behavioural field, and the many possibilities of clarifying and detecting living conditions for dyslexic persons in modern society put forth by sociological research, should not only be stimulating, but also of highest importance to future dyslexia research. Moreover, the behavioural and sociological fields should evaluate more the contributions of the biological and cognitive fields in their searches for insight and successful methods of intervention.

The second question was to what degree Lakatos philosophy of science would give a meta-perspective of the field of current dyslexia research. This question is easier to answer than the first one. By applying a meta-perspective, at least these authors have gained new insight in the different fields of dyslexia. Thus Lakatos' philosophy of research programmes became a useful framework for sorting out ideas. What perhaps was most surprising, was the way the differences between the sociological and the other three fields came forward. While the biological, cognitive and behavioural fields all define themselves as humanistic in that they clearly acknowledge the huge impact culture and environment have on their respective fields, the sociological field, at its outmost, takes an attitude of being incompatible with the other fields. This is done by defining only the sociological approach as humanistic and the other approaches as naturalistic, and by denying the existence of dyslexia.

However, the main idea left to us is that it would have been easier to apply the theories of Lakatos 10-20 years ago. Although the basic four fields have their own "hard cores", the intermingling and co-operation of fields, as can be seen in paper presentations and at conferences, is increasingly a prominent feature of dyslexia research today. Thus the critique of Feyerabend may have some relevance, at the same time as Lakatos' structure helps to find a system of storage that undoubtedly is clarifying. Also, his emphasis of the gradual building on "blocks" of earlier research (the hard core) is a way of giving less impact to Popper's claim of falsification, which can be discouraging to scientific enterprise. To what extent his ideas of avoiding "mobbing" within certain fields, have come true, is not easy to answer, but his theories support inclusion, rather than exclusion, of ideas. However, the gap between the "diagnostic" tradition and the "normalising" tradition within dyslexia research is an illustration of how there are still some mutual approaches between fields to be made.

For the moment presupposing that distinguishing between different research programmes is a legitimate and useful undertaking: To what extent is it possible, say desirable, to evaluate different research programmes in terms of progress and quality of research? Insofar as the programmes have overlapping interests and goals, as for instance those of the cognitive and the behavioural approaches, such comparisons are possible and sensible. The strong focus upon phonological deficits inherent in the cognitive approach may thus be evaluated from the point of view of behaviouristic approaches. But to the extent that the goals, methods and purposes of the programmes differ, the undertaking seems to make less sense. Thus, the sociological approach cannot be valued from the point of view of genetics. A possible explanation for this would be that Lakatos took his main examples from physics. In sciences with strong social components, this approach may be directly misleading, in that the goals and aims of these sciences cannot be easily made to fit the criteria of progress and growth of knowledge.

REFERENCES

Bakker, D. J. (1992). "Neuropsychological classification and treatment of dyslexia." *Journal of Learning Disabilities* **25**(2): 102-109.

Beaton, A. B. (2004). *Dyslexia, Reading and the Brain*. East Sussex, Psychology Press.

Behan, P. and N. Geschwind (1985). "Dyslexia, congenital anomalies, and immune disorders: The role of the fetal environment. Institute for Child Development Research Conference: Hope for a new neurology (1984, New York, New York)." *Annals of the New York Academy of Sciences* **457**: 13-18.

Boder, E. (1969). Developmental Dyslexia: A Diagnostic Screening Procedure Based on Readin and Spelling Patterns.

Boder, E. (1973). "Developmental dyslexia: A diagnostic approach based on three atypical reading-spelling patterns." *Developmental Medicine & Child Neurology* **15**: 663-687.

Chamers, A. F. (1982). *What is this thing called science?* St. Lucia, Open University Press.

Fagerheim, T., F. E. Tønnesen, et al. (1999). Exclusion of linkage to 1p, 6p and chromosome 15 in a large Norwegian family with dyslexia. *Dyslexia: Advances in Theory and Practice*. I. Lundberg, F. E. Tønnesen and I. Austad. Dordrecht, KLuwer Academic Publishers. **16**.

Feyerabend, P. (1975). *Against Method*. London, New York, Verso.

Fletcher, J., S. E. Shaywitz, et al. (1994). "Cognitive profiles of reading disability: Comparisons of discrepancy and low achievement definitions." *Journal of Educational Psychology* **86**(1): 6-23.

Frith, U. (1985). "The usefulness of the concept of unexpected reading failure: Comments on "Reading retardation revisited."" *British Journal of Developmental Psychology* **3**(1): 15-17.

Frith, U. (1997). Brain, Mind and Behaviour in dyslexia. *Dyslexia: Biology, Cognition and Intervention*. C. Hulme and M. J. Snowling. London, Whurr Publishers Ltd.

Frith, U. (1999). "Paradoxes in the Definition of Dyslexia." *Dyslexia* **5**: 192-214.

Galaburda, A. M. (1990). "The testosterone hypothesis: Assessment since Geschwind and Behan, 1982. 40th Annual Conference of the Orton Dyslexia Society (1989, Dallas, Texas)." *Annals of Dyslexia* **40**: 18-38.

Geschwind, N. (1979). "Asymmetries of the brain--new developments." *Bulletin of the Orton Society* **29**: 67-73.

Geschwind, N. and A. M. Galaburda (1985). "Cerebral lateralization: Biological mechanisms, associations, and pathology: III. A hypothesis and a program for research." *Archives of Neurology* **42**(7): 634-654.

Gjessing, H. J. (1977). *Lese- og skrivevansker. Dyslexi (Reading and writing impairments. Dyslexia)*. Bergen, Universitetsforlaget.

Gjessing, H. J. (1986). "Function analysis as a way of subgrouping the reading disabled: Clinical and statistical analyses." *Scandinavian Journal of Educational Research* **30**(2): 95-106.

Goswami, U. (1999). Dyslexia in Different Orthographies. *Dyslexia: Advances in Theory and Practice*. I. Lundberg, F. E. Tønnesen and I. Austad. Dordrecht, Kluwer Academic Publishers. **16**: 101-116.

Hagtvet, B. E., T. Helland, et al. (2005). Literacy acquisition in Norwegian. *Handbook of Orthography and Literacy*. R. M. Joshi and P. G. Aaron. Mahwah, N. J., Lawrence Erlbaum Associates.

Helland, T. and A. E. Asbjornsen (2003). "Visual-sequential and visuo-spatial skills in dyslexia: Variations according to language comprehension and mathematics skills." *Child Neuropsychology* **9**(3): 208-220.

Helland, T. and A. E. Asbjørnsen (2004). "Digit Span in Dyslexia: Variations According to Language Comprehension Abilities and Mathematics Skills." *Journal of Clinical & Experimental Neuropsychology* **26**(1): 31-42.

Helland, T. and R. Kaasa (2005). "Dyslexia in English as a second language." *Dyslexia* **11**: 41-60.

Kuhn, T. S. (1970). *The Structure of Scientific Revolutiona*. Chicago, University of Chicago Press.

Lakatos, I. (1970). *Criticism and the Growth of Knowledge*. New York, Cambridge University Press.

Lakatos, I. (1978). Mathematics, Science and Epistemology. *Philosophical Papers, Vol. II.* C. J. Worrall, G. New York, Cambridge University Press.

Landerl, K. (2003). Dyslexia in German-speaking children. *Dyslexia in different languages. Cross-linguistic comparisons.* N.Goulandris. London, Whurr publishers.: 15-32.

Livingstone, M. S., G. D. Rosen, et al. (1991). "Physiological and Anatomical Evidence for a Magnocellular Defect in Developmental Dyslexia." *Proceedings of the National Academy of Sciences of the United States of America* **88**(18): 7943-7947.

Lundberg, I., F. E. Tønnesen, et al., Eds. (1999). *Dyslexia: Advances in Theory and Practice.* Neuropsychology and Cognition. Dordrecht, Kluwer Academic Publishers.

Morgan, A. E. (1892). "A case of word-blindness." *British Medical Journal????* **2**: 1378.

Morton, J. and U. Frith (1995). Causal modeling: A structural approach to developmental psychopathology. *Developmental psychopathology, Vol. 1: Theory and methods. Wiley series on personality processes.* D. J. C. Dante Cicchetti, John Wiley & Sons, New York, NY, US: 357-390.

Nicolson, R. I. and A. J. Fawcett (1999). "Developmental Dyslexia: The role of the Cerebellum." *Dyslexia* **5**: 155-177.

Olson, R. K. (1999). Research on reading disabilities in the Colorado Learning Disabilities Research Center. *Dyslexia: Advances in theory and practice.* I. Lundberg, F. E. Tønnesen and I. Austad. Dordrecht, Kluwer Academic Press. **16**.

Paulesu, E., J.-F. Démonet, et al. (2001). "Dyslexia: Cultural Diversity and Biological Unity." *Science* **291**: 2165-2167.

Peer, L. and G. Reid (2000). *Multilingualism, Literacy and Dyslexia. A Challenge for Educators.* London, david Fulton Publishers.

Siegel, L. S. (1992). "An evaluation of the discrepancy definition of dyslexia." *Journal of Learning Disabilities* **25**(10): 618-629.

Solvang, P. (1995). "Dysleksidebatten - fra krise til forhandlingsperpektiv The discussion on dyslexia - from crisis to to a perpective of negotiations)." *Spesialpedagogikk* **6**.

Solvang, P. (1995). "Dysleksidebatten - to usammenlignbare posisjoner som begge er nødvendige? (The discussion on dyslexia - two incomparable positions that are both necessary?)." *Nordisk tidsskrift for spesialpedagogikk (Nordic Journal of special education)* **1**.

Solvang, P. (1998). " Den dyslektiske dominans. Lese- og skrivevansker som kunnskapsfelt i Norge." *Spesialpedagogikk* **8**.

Solvang, P. (1999). "Konstruktive kontroverser på feltet lese- og skrivevansker (Constructive controversies in the area of reading and writing impairments)." *Spesialpedagogikk* **2**.

Stein, J. F. (2000). "The neurobiology of reading difficulties." *Prostaglandins, Leukotrienes and Essential Fatty Acids* **0**: 1-8.

Stein, J. F. and V. Walsh (1997). "To see but not to read; the magnocellular theory of dyslexia." *Trends in Neuroscience* **20**(4): 147-52.

Tallal, P. (2000). Experimental studies of language learning impairments: From research to remediation. *Speech and language impairments in children: Causes, characteristics, intervention and outcome.* D. V. M. Bishop and L. B. Leonard. Hove, East Sussex, Psychology Press: 131-155.

The British Dyslexia Association (1998). The British Dyslexia Association Handbook. Reading, British Dyslexia Association.

The Orton Dyslexia Society (1994). A new definition of dyslexia, Bulletin of the Orton Dyslexia Society (now the International Dyslexia Association).

Tønnessen, F. E. (1995). "On defining "Dyslexia."" *Scandinavian Journal of Educational Research* **39**(2): 139-156. rights reserved).

Tønnessen, F. E. (1997). "How can we best define "Dyslexia"?" *Dyslexia* **3**: 78 - 92.

Uppstad, P. H. (2005). Language and Literacy. Some fundamental issues in research on reading and writing. *Department of Linguisitics and Phonetics*. Lund, Lund University: 193.

Vellutino, F. R. (1978). Visual Processing Deficiencies in Poor Readers: A Critique of Traditional Conceptualizations of the Etiology of Dyslexia.

Vellutino, F. R. (1979). *Dyslexia: Theory and Research*. Cambridge, Mass., MIT Press.

Vellutino, F. R. (1991). Dyslexia. *The emergence of language: Development and evolution: Readings from " Scientific American" magazine.* William S.-Y. Wang, W. H. Freeman & Co, Publishers, New York, NY, US: 159-170.

Wimmer, H. (1993). "Characteristics of developmental dyslexia in regular writing system." *Applied Psycholinguistics* **14**: 1-33.

In: Dyslexia in Children: New Research
Editor: Christopher B. Hayes, pp. 123-142

ISBN 1-59454-969-9
© 2006 Nova Science Publishers, Inc.

Chapter 7

IS A MAGNOCELLULAR DEFICIT THE CAUSE OF POOR FLANKED-LETTER IDENTIFICATION IN DEVELOPMENTAL DYSLEXIA?

David Omtzigt[1],*, Angélique W. Hendriks[2] and Herman H. J. Kolk[1]
[1] Nijmegen Institute for Cognition and Information,
Radboud University Nijmegen, the Netherlands
[2] Department of Special EducationBehavioural Science Institute,
Radboud University Nijmegen, the Netherlands

ABSTRACT

One hypothesis about the aetiology of developmental dyslexia is that it is partially caused by a deficit of the magnocellular pathway. Previous research (Omtzigt, Hendriks, and Kolk, 2002; Omtzigt and Hendriks, 2004) has indicated that the magnocellular system is in fact involved in the identification of flanked letters, the basic building blocks of text. Importantly, people with developmental dyslexia have indeed been found to experience problems with identifying flanked letters. Therefore, in the present study, it was tested directly whether the dyslexic problems with flanked-letter identification are due to a magnocellular deficit. We did this by comparing the single- and the flanked-letter-identification ability of university students with (N = 24) and without (N = 24) developmental dyslexia using pure colour contrast and pure luminance contrast between characters and background. The contrast manipulation can be considered a manipulation of magnocellular activity since the magnocellular system is relatively more sensitive to luminance modulation than is the parvocellular system, whereas the latter is the more sensitive to colour variation. In line with expectations, the dyslexic participants had difficulty identifying flanked letters and they also performed poorly in a coherent-motion task, presumably reflecting poor magnocellular function. The contrast manipulation,

* Corresponding author: David Omtzigt; E-mail: D.Omtzigt@lycos.nl. * Now at: School of Psychology, University of Leicester, Lancaster Road, Leicester LE1 9HN, United Kingdom.

however, failed to differentiate between the two groups. Possible explanations for these apparently discrepant findings are discussed.

Keywords: Magnocellular System; Visual attention; Isoluminance; Crowding; Reading; Dyslexia

INTRODUCTION

Developmental dyslexia is a common[1] reading disorder, of which the aetiology has been clarified only partially (e.g., Habib, 2000; Ramus et al., 2003; Snowling, 2000). Although it is generally accepted that a phonological deficit plays a fundamental role in the disorder, people with dyslexia have been demonstrated to perform poorly in a number of tasks that do not rely on phonological processes at all. Thus, the possibility exists that also other, non-phonological, impairments contribute to the disorder.

One of the areas outside the phonological domain where people with dyslexia have demonstrated poorer performance is the visual area. Anatomical, physiological, and psychophysical data have led to the belief that the magnocellular (but not the parvocellular) subsystem of the retino-geniculo-cortical pathway is affected in dyslexic individuals, and that this is one of the factors contributing to the reading problems (e.g., Cornelissen, Richardson, Mason, Fowler, and Stein, 1995; Demb, Boynton, Best, and Heeger, 1998; Eden et al., 1996; Livingstone, Rosen, Drislane, and Galaburda, 1991; Slaghuis and Lovegrove, 1985; Stein and Walsh, 1997; Steinman, Steinman, and Garzia, 1998; Vidyasagar, 1999; Witton et al., 1998), although this belief is not without its critics (e.g., Amitay, Ben-Yehudah, Banai, and Ahissar, 2002; Farrag, Khedr, and Abel-Naser, 2002; Hill and Raymond, 2002; Ramus et al., 2003; Raymond and Sorensen, 1998; Skottun, 2000; Stuart, McAnally, and Castles, 2001). One of the ways in which a magnocellular deficit has been hypothesised to impair reading is through a deficit in the attentional system (e.g., Stein and Walsh, 1997; Steinman et al., 1998; Vidyasagar, 1999). This can be motivated by the fact that there is strong magnocellular input into the dorsal ('where') stream (e.g., Milner and Goodale, 1995), which culminates in parietal cortex, an important area in the allocation of attention (Maunsell, 1992; Milner and Goodale, 1995; Ungerleider and Haxby, 1994).

There is in fact a large body of evidence pointing to an attentional anomaly in people with dyslexia. For instance, dyslexic readers have been found to exhibit impaired focusing (e.g., Facoetti, Paganoni, Turatto, Marzola, and Mascetti, 2000) and shifting (e.g., Facoetti et al., 2000; Hari and Renvall, 2001; Steinman et al., 1998) of attention, as well as hemifield-specific abnormalities (e.g., Facoetti and Turatto, 2000; Hari, Renvall, and Tanskanen, 2001). The question thus arises as to how an attention deficit could affect reading.

As a first possibility, it could have a negative effect on letter identification. It is well known that stimuli that are flanked by other stimuli are more difficult to identify than are stimuli that appear alone (often termed 'crowding'). Various studies have shown a role of attentional factors in processing flanked stimuli (Facoetti, 2001; Huckauf and Heller, 2002; Intriligator and Cavanagh, 2001; Leat, Li, and Epp, 1999; Shiu and Pashler, 1995;

---

[1] About 7% of the 9 to 11-year-old children in the Netherlands are dyslexic (school year 2001/2002; source: Centraal Bureau voor de Statistiek, Voorburg/Heerlen, the Netherlands).

Strasburger, Harvey Jr., and Rentschler, 1991; Wolford and Chambers, 1983). Thus, it is possible that the attentional anomaly in people with developmental dyslexia affects the identification of information surrounded by other information, in particular the identification of the letters in text. This idea is supported by a variety of studies. For instance, dyslexic individuals have been found to perform less well than normal readers in visual-search tasks (e.g., Facoetti et al., 2000; Vidyasagar and Pammer, 1999) and to demonstrate atypical compatibility effects in Eriksen-type flanker tasks (Facoetti and Turatto, 2000; Klein and D'Entremont, 1999). Most pertinently, dyslexic individuals have indeed been found to have difficulties in identifying letters flanked by other letters (Atkinson, 1991, 1993; Bouma and Legein, 1977, 1980) and words flanked by other words (Spinelli, De Luca, Judica, and Zoccolotti, 2002).

A second possibility of an attention deficit affecting reading is that it could impair the correct positioning of the letters within words. During the fixation periods of reading, attention is thought to be directed in a rapid, sequential manner across the letters in a text (Vidyasagar, 1999). Thus, if the attentional spotlight does not move appropriately, the order of letters and letter clusters could become distorted. Indeed, letter-ordering problems are often mentioned as one of the main characteristics of dyslexia (e.g., Boder, 1973; Orton, 1937; Stein, 2003).

A third possibility of an attention deficit affecting reading is that it could interfere with the execution of saccadic eye movements. A shift of attention always precedes a saccade (e.g., Deubel and Schneider, 1996; McPeek, Maljkovic, and Nakayama, 1999; Shepherd, Findlay, and Hockey, 1986). Thus, if the shifting of attention is somehow disrupted, saccades may be disrupted as well, which would be detrimental to the reading process. Indeed, saccadic anomalies have been reported in dyslexic readers (e.g., Rayner, 1998).

The present study focuses on the first of these three possible detrimental effects of magnocellular dysfunction on attention in reading. We presented the letter-naming task from a previous study of ours (Omtzigt, Hendriks, and Kolk, 2002), which had been carried out with normal readers only, both to normally reading and to dyslexic participants. Importantly, this task was based on the earlier mentioned letter-naming task demonstrating poor flanked-letter identification in dyslexic individuals (Bouma and Legein, 1977, 1980). However, unlike the original task of Bouma and Legein (1977, 1980), which contained one stimulus-background contrast only, we used colour contrast and weak luminance contrast between characters and background: Colour contrast is known to trigger parvocellular activity better than magnocellular activity, whereas for weak levels of luminance contrast, the reverse is true (Livingstone and Hubel, 1988). Therefore, colour versus luminance contrast can be used as a manipulation of magnocellular activity. As such, it can simulate a comparison between normal and impaired magnocellular function, and probably, indirectly, between a normal and an impaired attentional system.

In our previous study (Omtzigt et al., 2002), we found that colour contrast and weak luminance contrast led to similar naming performance for the presentation of single letters, whereas colour contrast led to worse naming performance than luminance contrast for the presentation of flanked letters. This contrast × stimulus interaction was interpreted as evidence for a role of the magnocellular system in flanked-letter identification, and, therefore, possibly, in the allocation of attention. Support for this latter conclusion was obtained in a follow-up study with an explicit attention-cueing manipulation (Omtzigt and Hendriks, 2004): the interaction appeared only in conditions where participants did not receive information about stimulus location. Thus, with respect to the present study, if poor magnocellular function does indeed play a role in the flanked-letter-identification impairment in developmental dyslexia, one would expect the interaction to be smaller for the dyslexic readers, because an increase of magnocellular input during luminance-contrast relative to colour-contrast presentation may be expected to be less effective for a magnocellular system that is deficient (e.g., if in dyslexic readers magnocellular activity cannot be processed at all, a manipulation of magnocellular activity should have no effect).

To assess magnocellular function independently of the letter-naming task, a coherent-motion task was administered. People with developmental dyslexia usually score more poorly on this task than normal readers (e.g., Cornelissen et al., 1995; Hansen, Stein, Orde, Winter, and Talcott, 2001; Pammer and Wheatley, 2001; Ridder III, Borsting, and Banton, 2001; Slaghuis and Ryan, 1999; Witton et al., 1998; but see, e.g., Amitay et al., 2002; Ramus et al., 2003). It should be noted, though, that although the coherent-motion task is often considered a measure of magnocellular activity, it could also reflect the functioning of dorsal extrastriate areas involved in the segmentation and/or integration of motion signals (e.g., Hill and Raymond, 2002; Raymond and Sorensen, 1998) or that of the parietal cortex itself, since motion perception has been shown to be modulated by attention (Raymond, 2000).

Finally, all participants were given a word-reading task, a nonword-reading task, a difficult phonological task, and a non-verbal IQ test (see Method section for details), only the first three of which should yield significantly worse performance for the dyslexic than for the normally reading participants.

METHOD

Participants

Twenty-four dyslexic and 24 non-dyslexic students from Radboud University Nijmegen took part in the experiment. In each group, there were 12 males and 12 females. For the dyslexic group, age ranged from 20 to 30, with a median of 23; for the non-dyslexic group, age ranged from 18 to 29, with a median of 22.5. The participants were paid or given course credit for their participation. All reported that they had normal or corrected-to-normal vision including normal colour vision, as well as normal hearing. The dyslexic students had all been officially diagnosed as dyslexic; they were recruited via the disability office of the university. The non-dyslexic students were non-dyslexic by self-report.

Materials, Design, Procedure, and Data-Analysis

All participants were tested on the six tasks in the following order: coherent-motion task, letter-identification task, word-reading task, nonword-reading task, phonological task, and non-verbal IQ test. The whole session took about one hour.

Coherent-Motion Task

The coherent-motion stimuli were generated by a Pentium-III PC and presented on a Philips Brilliance 107P monitor with B22 phosphor. The refresh rate of the screen was 70 Hz and the resolution was 800×600 pixels. The coherent-motion stimuli and the threshold determination were similar to those used by Cornelissen, Hansen, Hutton, Evangelinou, and Stein (1998). Differently from Cornelissen et al.'s (1998) stimuli, however, in which two juxtaposed patches with dots were presented, one of which contained the coherent motion, in the present study we used only one (centrally presented) patch that always contained coherent motion, either in the horizontal or in the vertical dimension. This was done to minimise the possibility that the expected coherent-motion-threshold difference between the dyslexic and the control group was due to a possibly different viewing strategy, which might arise in the case of two patches (sequential vs. simultaneous viewing).

The patch contained 300 white dots against a dark background that was indistinguishable from the rest of the screen. With the lights out, the luminance of the dots was 108.3 cd/m^2 and the luminance of the background was 0.53 cd/m^2, as measured with a Spectra Pritchard 1980A-CD photometer using a photopic filter, yielding a Michelson contrast of 99%. Viewed from a distance of 60 cm, the patch subtended 8.8 by 12.4 degrees, and each individual dot was 0.076 by 0.074 degrees wide (i.e., 2×2 pixels). Individual dots were visible for about 29 ms (i.e., two frames), after which a certain percentage of the dots were displaced systematically either horizontally by 0.46 degrees or vertically by 0.45 degrees (the different numbers are due to the slightly different pixel sizes in the horizontal and the vertical dimensions) giving coherent motion with a speed of 15.7 deg/s or 15.4 deg/s, respectively; the remaining dots were displaced to random locations within the patch. Dots were visible in their new locations for another 29 ms. Then, all the dots were displaced randomly and the procedure started anew.[2] Coherent dots moved in the same direction ten times in succession, after which the direction was reversed. There were three such reversals. Total stimulus duration was thus 2286 ms (i.e., $2 \times 2 \times 10 \times 4$ frames). Whether the coherent dots moved horizontally or vertically was determined on a random basis, as was the direction of the initial movement (left or right, or up or down). The participants keyed in their response after the stimulus had disappeared from the screen. There was no time pressure.

For the threshold determination, a two-alternative forced-choice 1-up-1-down staircase procedure was used. For each correct response, the percentage of coherently moving dots was reduced by a factor of 1.122; for each incorrect response, the percentage was increased by a factor of 1.412. At the beginning of the staircase, 90% of the dots moved coherently. After the direction of the staircase had reversed ten times, the threshold was calculated. The first two reversals were discarded and of the remaining eight the geometric mean was calculated, which was taken as the threshold for the run in question. Three threshold determinations were carried out for each participant, of which the first was discarded for practice reasons. Of the remaining two, the arithmetic mean was taken as the participant's final score.

---

[2] There were two unintended differences with the stimuli used in Cornelissen et al. (1998). First, in the latter study, the not coherently moving dots moved about in a Brownian manner, that is, they were displaced a fixed distance (the same distance as the coherently moving dots) from their initial location with random angle, instead of being displaced completely randomly. Second, in Cornelissen et al.'s (1998) study, coherent motion was defined every 29 ms instead of only once every 58 ms as in the present study. These unintended differences may have rendered the present coherent-motion stimuli suboptimal for measuring a magnocellular deficit in developmental dyslexia (see also the Results section).

Letter-Identification Task

This task was virtually identical to the letter-identification task used in Omtzigt et al. (2002). Stimuli were generated by an Apple Power Macintosh 7200/90 and presented on an Apple Multiple Scan 15" Display (M2978) with aluminised P22 medium-short persistence phosphor. The CIE co-ordinates of the phosphors were as follows: for red, x = 0.610, y = 0.342; for green, x = 0.298, y = 0.588; for blue, x = 0.151, y = 0.064. The refresh rate of the screen was 66.7 Hz. Screen resolution was 640 × 480 pixels, and the computer was running in 256-colour mode. Luminance and the contrast of the monitor were set at their maximum values.

In each condition and for each participant, all the letters of the Dutch alphabet (which is identical to the English alphabet) were presented except the letters x, q, and y (because these are very infrequent in the Dutch language), and with the letters a, e, i, o, and u presented more than once, giving 32 letter presentations per condition in total. Participants were not informed about the selection of the letters and the number of times they would appear. All letters were presented in a bold Geneva font of 31 points. Given the distance of the participants to the monitor (80 cm), this amounted to approximately 0.4 degrees of visual angle per letter. In the flanked-letter conditions, each letter was flanked by two *x*s (one to the left and one to the right) that were positioned such that the distance between the centres of two adjacent letters was approximately 0.5 degrees. The background was yellow throughout the experiment. With the lights out, the luminance level of the background was 13.0 cd/m^2, as measured with a Spectra Pritchard 1980A-CD photometer using a photopic filter. In the luminance-contrast conditions, targets and distracters differed from the background only with respect to their luminance: They were slightly above the background level (13.7 cd/m^2), resulting in a Michelson contrast of 2.6%. In the colour-contrast conditions, targets and distracters had a green appearance (the RGB values were usually within the range of (0.074, 0.227, 0) to (0.078, 0.242, 0)) and their luminance was set by means of heterochromatic flicker photometry such that virtually no luminance contrast remained between characters and background. The flickering stimulus was a centrally presented disk subtending approximately 2.5 degrees of visual angle against a dark background. The disk flickered continuously alternating the colour contrast's fore- and background colour at a rate of 11.1 Hz. The luminance level of the foreground was adjusted manually by the experimenter until a level was found for which the participant judged the flicker to be minimal, after which it was recorded for use in the letter-naming experiment.

There were three within-subject manipulations: contrast between letters and background (colour vs. luminance), stimulus (flanked letters vs. single letters), and location of letter presentation (1° to the left of fixation, central, or 1° to the right of fixation). Location varied randomly from trial to trial with the restrictions that all locations were used equally often in each block and that the same location was not used for more than three trials in a row. Contrast and stimulus remained constant during blocks and were counterbalanced across and within participants. There were 16 blocks in total, and there were four different block orders across participants. Each block contained 24 stimuli. Letter-identity order was randomised but with the restriction that consecutive letter identities were different. For each participant in the dyslexic group, there was one participant in the control group whothat received exactly the same stimulus list (in every respect).

Prior to the start of the letter-identification experiment, the flicker-photometry procedure was carried out. The actual letter-identification experiment began with one block of practice trials containing two occurrences of every condition. Before each letter presentation, a central fixation mark appeared for 210 ms, which consisted of two vertical dashes one above the other just outside the area where a centrally presented letter stimulus would appear. It had the same yellow colour as the background but a somewhat higher level of luminance. The fixation stimulus disappeared 300 ms before the presentation of the letter. Letter-stimulus duration was 105 ms. Participants were instructed to name the target letter as quickly as possible and to make a guess in case they could not determine which letter had been presented. The start of the participants' vocal responses was picked up by means of a microphone attached to a headphones (which served no purpose other than to keep the microphone close to the participants' mouths) connected to a voice-key, which was integrated in the button-box that was used for the task. The inter-trial interval started automatically after a response had been made (or 7500 ms after letter-presentation initiation if no response had been detected) and lasted 1500 ms. During this interval, the screen remained yellow. There were breaks between all sixteen stimulus blocks.

Dependent variables were the mean reaction time (RT) and the percentage of errors. Before calculation of these measures, 8.9% of the data had to be discarded. First, trials without or with an ambiguous response, trials with voice-key failure, and trials with an RT of less than 300 ms were removed. Then, for the remaining data, for each of the conditions of every participant, the mean RT was determined. All responses that were more than two standard deviations slower or faster than their corresponding mean RT value were considered to be outliers and therefore discarded. Subsequently, the mean RT values were calculated anew and percentages of errors were determined. These new mean RT values and the error percentages were finally used in the statistical analyses to be reported in the Results section.

Reading Tasks

All participants were tested with Form A of the Een-Minuut-Test [One-Minute-Test] (Brus and Voeten, 1999), a Dutch paper-based word-reading test composed of 116 single words, and with Form A of the De Klepel (Van den Bos, Lutje Spelberg, Scheepsma, and De Vries, 1999), a Dutch paper-based nonword-reading test containing 116 items as well, which were constructed on the basis of the items of Form A of the Een-Minuut-Test. The participants received the standard one minute for the word-reading test and the standard two minutes for the nonword-reading test to read as many words or nonwords correctly as they could. The number of correct responses was used as the dependent variable.

Phonological Task

To take the possibility into account that the adult dyslexic participants might haved obtained relatively good phonological skills, a difficult phoneme-manipulation task was created. Forty Dutch-legal nonwords were constructed which were still Dutch-legal nonwords if all of their phonemes were put in the reversed order (e.g., /flon/ and /nolf/). All nonwords were monosyllabic, and the beginning, as well as the final phoneme, was always a consonant. The nonwords were digitally recorded for standardised administration; they were spoken by a female speaker with a standard Dutch accent. The participants received the nonwords via headphones.

In each trial, one nonword was presented. The participants had to repeat the nonword and then produce the 'phoneme-reversed' version, both verbally. The instruction was to be as fast and as accurate as possible, and there was a maximum of two minutes to do the task. Two practice items preceded the experimental list. Whenever a participant needed to hear a nonword again, they could press a button for a repetition. Each new stimulus presentation was initiated by the participants themselves.

The number of correct responses was used as the dependent variable. Both the original and the phoneme-reversed version of a nonword had to be right in order for the response to be counted as correct. (Note: the original version was only occasionally mispronounced incorrectly: 3.2% of the trials of the dyslexic and 4.3% of the trials of the normally reading participants.)

Non-Verbal IQ Test

A subtest ('Legkaart') of the Groninger Intelligentie Test (Luteijn and Van der Ploeg, 1983), a Dutch intelligence test, was used to measure the participants' non-verbal IQ. In this subtest, it should be indicated which out of several drawn shapes fit together to form a larger figure (similar to the game of Tangram). There were 20 different puzzles. The test's official timing was adjusted slightly to have the entire experimental session finished within about an hour, leaving one minute per puzzle. If participants had not responded within 50 seconds, they were warned of their nearly running out of time. The participants could proceed to the next puzzle before time was up, but they could not return to a previous puzzle. There were two practice puzzles at the beginning of the test. The number of correct responses was taken as the dependent variable.

RESULTS

To verify the classification of participants into dyslexic and non-dyslexic readers, their scores on the word- and the nonword-reading task, the phonological task, and the non-verbal IQ-test were compared. The dyslexics as a group performed considerably more poorly than did the control group on word reading and nonword reading [88.9 vs. 111.1 words read correctly, $t(29.78) = 6.44$, $p < .001$,[3] one-tailed; 81.8 vs. 108.0 nonwords read correctly, $t(27.53) = 6.06$, $p < .001$, one-tailed; note that the degrees of freedom had to be adjusted due to unequal variances] and on the phonological task [17.8 vs. 25.9 correct nonword reversals, $t(46) = 4.47$, $p < .001$, one-tailed]. By contrast, the dyslexic readers were as good as the normal readers on the intelligence test [13.8 vs. 14.0 correct solutions, $t(46) = 0.33$, ns]. These results confirm the classification of our participants into dyslexic and non-dyslexic readers.

---

[3] Throughout the chapter, when a specific direction of an effect had been hypothesised, the one-tailed p value is given (which is also indicated as such). Importantly, note that also in the context of ANOVAs the use of one-tailed p values is legitimate: If an effect (main or interaction) involves only two-level factors, the F test is algebraically equivalent to a t test (see also Ley, 1979). Whenever a one-tailed p value is used without an explicit prediction having been formulated, the prediction followed the results of our previous study (Omtzigt et al., 2002).

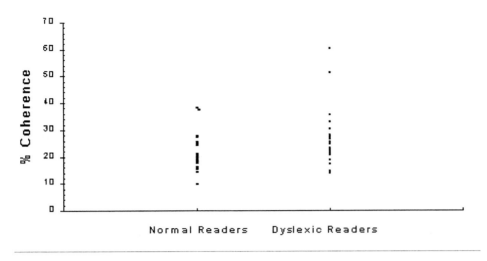

Figure 1. Individual performance in the coherent-motion task (percentage coherence threshold) for the normal and the dyslexic readers separately.

For the coherent-motion task, the dyslexics needed a significantly larger percentage of coherently moving dots to perceive the coherent motion than did the controls [26.0% versus 21.1%, $t(46) = 1.92$, $p < .05$, one-tailed] (see Figure 1). This finding is in agreement with what is usually found (e.g., Cornelissen et al., 1995; Hansen, Stein, Orde, Winter, and Talcott, 2001; Pammer and Wheatley, 2001; Ridder III, Borsting, and Banton, 2001; Slaghuis and Ryan, 1999; Witton et al., 1998) and suggests that our dyslexic-participant group have impaired magnocellular function. However, as can also be seen in Figure 1, there is substantial overlap between the two groups. Although large overlap between normal and dyslexic readers is not uncommon in the coherent-motion task, it does suggest that the magnocellular deficit in the present dyslexic group is small, so that it might prove difficult to find group effects in the letter-identification task. Alternatively, it might be the case that our coherent-motion task was not optimal for measuring a magnocellular deficit (see also Footnote 2).

For the letter-identification task, a $2 \times 2 \times 2 \times 3$ (group × contrast × stimulus × location) repeated-measures multivariate analysis of variance was conducted, with group as a between-subjects factor, on the RTs and on the error scores. All four main effects were significant in both the RT and the error-score analysis: The dyslexic readers were slower and less accurate than were the non-dyslexic readers [$F(1, 46) = 5.90$, $p < .01$, one-tailed, for RTs; $F(1, 46) = 6.83$, $p < .01$, one-tailed, for error scores]; colour contrast led to slower and less accurate responses than did luminance contrast [$F(1, 46) = 12.30$, $p < .01$, for RTs; $F(1, 46) = 19.85$, $p < .001$, for error scores]; the flanked letters were responded to more slowly and less accurately than were the single letters [$F(1, 46) = 115.72$, $p < .001$, one-tailed, for RTs; $F(1, 46) = 186.65$, $p < .001$, one-tailed, for error scores]; and performance depended on the location of letter presentation [$F(2, 45) = 52.64$, $p < .001$, for RTs; $F(2, 45) = 107.22$, $p < .001$, for error scores], with the non-central letters being more difficult than the central letters [$F(1, 46) = 84.51$, $p < .001$, one-tailed, for RTs; $F(1, 46) = 218.74$, $p < .001$, one-tailed, for error scores] and letter presentations to the left and right being equally difficult [$F(1, 46) = 1.70$, ns, for RTs; $F(1, 46) = 0.21$, ns, for error scores]. See Figure 2 for the effects of group, contrast, and stimulus. The main effect of group replicates the findings of Bouma and Legein

(1977, 1980), and the main effects of stimulus and location are also in accordance with Bouma and Legein's findings (1977, 1980), as well as with our own previous findings (Omtzigt et al., 2002). The main effect of contrast was different from our previous study in that here colour contrast was less adequate than luminance contrast not only for flanked [$F(1, 46) = 23.54, p < .001$, for RTs; $F(1, 46) = 27.04, p < .001$, for error scores] but also for single letters [$F(1, 46) = 1.89, ns$, for RTs; $F(1, 46) = 5.37, p < .05$, for error scores]. However, this was probably due to slightly changed colour appearances relative to those in our previous study (Omtzigt et al., 2002). Moreover, the interaction of contrast with stimulus (see below) was still significant, so that the present single-letter contrast data do not disqualify the present (or the previous) results.

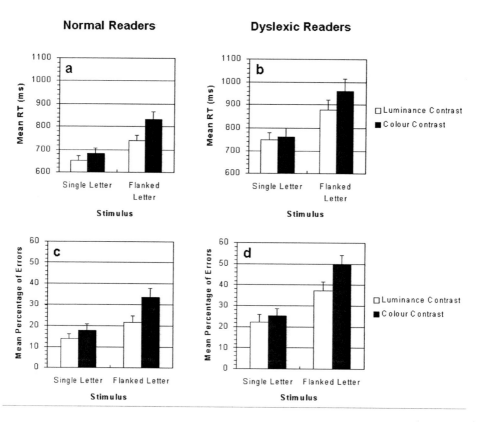

Figure 2. Mean naming performance with standard error as a function of contrast and stimulus averaged across location) in the letter-identification task for: (a) reaction time (RT) and the normal readers; (b) reaction time (RT) and the dyslexic readers; (c) percentage of errors and the normal readers; (d) percentage of errors and the dyslexic readers.

Regarding the interactions that did not include the group factor, nearly all effects were significant, thereby essentially replicating the results of our previous study (Omtzigt et al., 2002). The effect of contrast × stimulus [$F(1, 46) = 26.81, p < .001$, one-tailed, for RTs; $F(1, 46) = 21.87, p < .001$, one-tailed, for error scores] was that colour-contrast performance was worse than luminance-contrast performance for the flanked letters in particular. This result was the basic finding of our previous study (Omtzigt et al., 2002), and was interpreted as evidence for the importance of magnocellular input to the identification of flanked letters.

Contrast × location [$F(2, 45) = 6.51, p < .01$, for RTs; $F(2, 45) = 10.51, p < .001$, for error scores] and stimulus × location [$F(2, 45) = 42.27, p < .001$, for RTs; $F(2, 45) = 44.87, p < .001$, for error scores] yielded that colour-contrast presentation and flanked letters were particularly more difficult for non-central presentations, respectively.

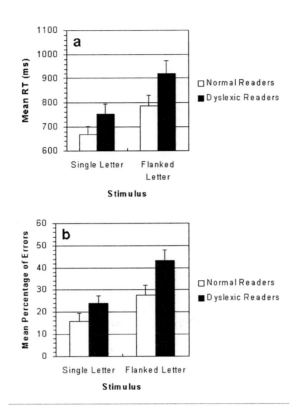

Figure 3. Mean naming performance with standard error as a function of participant group and stimulus (averaged across contrast and location) in the letter-identification task for: (a) reaction time (RT); (b) percentage of errors.

Regarding the interactions that did include the group factor, only the interaction of group × stimulus was significant [$F(1, 46) = 3.71, p < .05$, one-tailed, for RTs; $F(1, 46) = 11.40, p < .001$, one-tailed, for error scores]: The dyslexic participants were poorer than the controls at identifying the single letters [$F(1, 46) = 4.88, p < .05$, one-tailed, for RTs; $F(1, 46) = 4.07, p < .05$, one-tailed, for error scores], but they were particularly poor at identifying the flanked target letters [$F(1, 46) = 6.15, p < .01$, one-tailed, for RTs; $F(1, 46) = 8.79, p < .01$, one-tailed, for error scores]; see Figure 3. This result is very important, because it essentially replicates the finding of Bouma and Legein (1977, 1980) of poor flanked-letter identification in dyslexic readers, which we hypothesised could be caused by poor a magnocellular deficitfunction. However, the predicted interaction of group × contrast × stimulus, which was crucial to the hypothesis that magnocellular dysfunction actually underlies poor flanked-letter identification, turned out not to be significant [$F(1, 46) = 0.17, ns$, for RTs; $F(1, 46) = 0.14, ns$, for error scores] (see Figure 2).

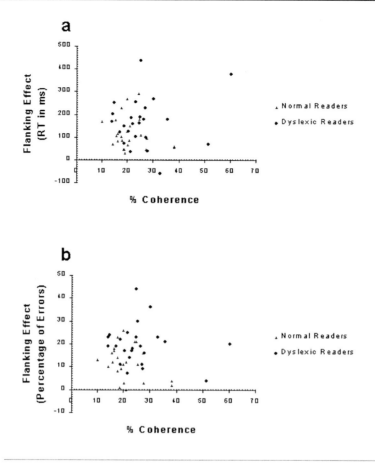

Figure 4. Scatter diagram for: (a) flanking effect expressed in RT by performance in the coherent-motion task (percentage coherence threshold) for the normal and the dyslexic readers; (b) flanking effect expressed in percentage of errors by performance in the coherent-motion task (percentage coherence threshold) for the normal and the dyslexic readers.

To investigate the relationship between magnocellular function and letter identification also in a different way, in Figure 4, a scatter diagram has been plotted for performance in the coherent motion task and the flanking effect (i.e., the difference in naming performance between the flanked letters and the single letters, averaged across contrast and location), for RTs (Figure 4a) and error scores (Figure 4b). As can be seen, no correlation is present, not for the group of dyslexic readers [$r = .14$, *ns*, for RTs; $r = -.14$, *ns*, for error scores], not for the group of normal readers [$r = -.18$, *ns*, for RTs; $r = -.32$, *ns*, for error scores], and also not for the two participant groups together [$r = .12$, *ns*, for RTs; $r = -.05$, *ns*, for error scores]. However, because there was such a large overlap between the two participant groups on the coherent-motion task, this was also to be expected.

CONCLUSION

Similar to previous studies (Bouma and Legein, 1977, 1980), we found the letter-identification ability of people with developmental dyslexia to suffer more from the presence of flanking *"letters"* than that of normal readers. Also like previous research (e.g., Cornelissen, et al., 1995; Hansen et al., 2001; Pammer and Wheatley, 2001; Ridder III et al., 2001; Slaghuis and Ryan, 1999; Witton et al., 1998), we found dyslexic readers to perform relatively poorly in a coherent-motion task, presumably reflecting a poorly functioning magnocellular system. Further, as was the case in our previous study (Omtzigt et al., 2002), we obtained a significant interaction of contrast × stimulus, with colour contrast relatively unsuited for the identification of flanked letters, suggesting that magnocellular input was important to flanked-letter identification. Thus, three major conditions had been satisfied for a successful verification of the hypothesis that poor magnocellular function causes poor flanked-letter identification in developmental dyslexia. Nevertheless, the contrast-by-stimulus interaction turned out to be similar for the dyslexic and the non-dyslexic readers. This seems to suggest that the flanked-letter-identification impairment was *not* due to abnormal magnocellular function.

However, this conclusion is perhaps premature. First, the specific experimental circumstances may have allowed the dyslexic readers to profit relatively more from magnocellular information during flanked-letter identification, despite their lower-functioning magnocellular system, thus *counteracting* the predicted second-order interaction of group × contrast × stimulus. Paradoxically, dyslexics' different (slower) attentional system (e.g., Facoetti et al., 2003; Hari and Renvall, 2001; Steinman et al., 1997) may have been responsible for this. In a previous study of ours (Omtzigt and Hendriks, 2004), it was found that if attention is cued to the correct or to the incorrect location of subsequent stimulus presentation, the interaction of contrast × stimulus disappears, suggesting that magnocellular information loses its importance or usability during flanked-letter identification. Although in the present study attention was not cued directly, some inadvertent cueing may have arisen in response to the fixation stimulus. If it was the case that this cueing effect was less strong for the dyslexic readers, magnocellular information may have come to be used relatively more extensively by these readers.

Second, the power of the experimental design may not have been high enough to reveal a significant second-order interaction of group × contrast × stimulus. If the true interaction of contrast × stimulus was indeed smaller for the dyslexic participants, let us say at a level of half the true interaction for the non-dyslexic participants, there was a probability of only around 30% of actually finding a significantly smaller interaction for the dyslexic readers (calculated under the assumption that the present mean of the normal readers and the standard deviations of both reader groups represented the true values), both for reaction times and for error scores. Also, the 95%-confidence interval for the observed group difference of the interaction included both the zero difference of the null-hypothesis and the 50% difference of the alternative hypothesis. To increase power, two important possibilities exist: increasing the total number of participants, or finding dyslexic participants for whom the interaction of contrast × stimulus could be expected to be especially small. As shown in the Results section, there was large overlap between the two participant groups on the coherent-motion task, possibly reflecting a small magnocellular deficit in the dyslexic readers (who were all university students). Inclusion of a large number of truly poor coherent-motion perceivers in the latter group could therefore significantly increase the probability of finding a significant group × contrast × stimulus interaction.

A previous study comparing dyslexic and normal readers on colour and luminance contrast in a reading task did already find an interaction involving reader group and contrast (O'Brien, 1996/1997). The participants in this study were required to read sentences from a computer display that were presented either as a whole or word-by-word (using the rapid-serial-visual-presentation technique) thus obviating saccadic eye movements. In both presentation conditions, the normal readers read significantly worse with colour contrast than with luminance contrast, whereas no significant performance difference between contrasts was observed for the dyslexic readers. Such an outcome can be explained if it was the case that the dyslexics could not make normal use of their magnocellular system so that a reduction of magnocellular input as happened under colour contrast did not harm their reading. Moreover, the group-by-contrast interaction was the same during normal and rapid-serial-visual presentation. This is an important finding because it suggests that the group-by-contrast interaction reflected discrepant magnocellular-system-related activity in relation to subprocesses of reading that were unrelated to the execution of saccades. Thus, O'Brien's (1996/1997) group-by-contrast interaction could imply dysfunction of exactly the same subprocesses of reading as studied here, since the critical contrast-by-stimulus interaction in the present study was most likely unrelated to the execution of saccades.

Strong evidence for the role of attention , and, hence, possibly the magnocellular system, in dyslexics' flanked-letter-identification problems comes from recent studies using a variant of the Eriksen flanker task (see, e.g., Eriksen and Eriksen, 1974). In such a task, a target is flanked by a number of distracters that are or are not response-compatible with the target. Participants are instructed to press one of two buttons depending on the target's identity (two-alternative forced choice). Flankers that are response-compatible may lead to better task performance, whereas flankers that are response-incompatible may lead to worse task performance; the performance difference between response-incompatible and response-compatible trials is defined as the compatibility effect. Using this methodology, Facoetti and Turatto (2000) observed that in a flanker task with (para)foveally presented (arrow) symbols dyslexic readers exhibited a stronger compatibility effect in their right visual field and a smaller compatibility effect in their left visual field compared with normal readers. Klein and D'Entremont (1999) presented digits within the foveal area and found that their dyslexic participants showed a compatibility effect that was virtually independent of the distance between the flankers and the target, whereas their normally reading participants showed the standard decrease in the compatibility effect for increasing distance. Thus, it was concluded that dyslexic readers have a problem with the suppression of information flanking the target (at least in their right visual field) (Facoetti and Turatto, 2000; Klein and D'Entremont, 1999). With respect to its relationship with reading, it has been hypothesised that the suppression problem may lead to difficulties focussing attention on the relevant units of text, which could affect the acquisition of orthographic principles and grapheme-phoneme-correspondence rules as well as their successful application once they have been mastered (Klein and D'Entremont, 1999). Importantly, there is evidence that the dyslexic readers who are poor at reading nonwords (which requires extensive use of the grapheme-phoneme-correspondence rules) are precisely those readers that are the most likely to have a magnocellular deficit (Borsting et al.,

1996; Cestnick and Coltheart, 1999; Slaghuis and Ryan, 1999; Ridder III, Borsting, Cooper, McNeel, and Huang, 1997; however, see Ridder III et al., 2001).

If it is indeed the case that a magnocellular deficit is responsible for the attentional difficulties in dyslexic readers, it may be interesting to speculate as to the precise characteristics of this deficit. One possibility is that the magnocellular system of dyslexic readers provides coarser input for the attentional-selection system than is the case in normal readers. It is conceivable that with such a magnocellular system, it is very difficult if not impossible to attend to small portions of the visual field, thus preventing the selection of small text units of text. Consistent with this, Talcott, Hansen, Assoku, and Stein (2000) found that poor performance of dyslexic readers in the coherent-motion task disappeared if the total number of dots was increased, possibly indicating spatial undersampling regarding motion-sensitive (and, hence, magnocellular-driven) mechanisms. Importantly, the speculation that the magnocellular system in dyslexic readers may provide less detailed visual information than is the case in normal readers may also play a role in resolving part of the controversy regarding contrast-sensitivity measurements. It has been argued that if a magnocellular deficit is present in dyslexic people, it should yield a selective insensitivity to low spatial frequencies of less than 1.5 cycles/deg because these are the frequencies that predominantly activate the magnocellular system. Paradoxically, however, such an outcome has been rarely obtained (see Skottun, 2000, for a review). Part of the solution could be that the spatial frequencies that are of relevance to the magnocellular system during reading and of which the perception is affected in dyslexic individuals are in the range between 1.5 and 10 cycles/deg, where the parvocellular system predominates perception but where the magnocellular system is also active for supra-threshold levels of contrast (see Chase, Ashourzadeh, Kelly, Monfette, and Kinsey, 2003, for a discussion of the spatial frequencies used during reading and their visibility to the magno- and parvocellular pathways). A magnocellular deficit could thus remain undetected.

Although its relationship with impaired magnocellular function could not be established in the present study, the finding that dyslexic university students exhibit a flanked-letter-identification impairment is interesting in its own right. It extends the data of Bouma and Legein (1977, 1980), who did their research with primary-school-age children, and it therefore suggests that the flanked-letter-identification impairment is a basic characteristic of dyslexia that may affect dyslexics' reading behaviour throughout their lives. Importantly, calculation of the correlation coefficients between the flanking effect (the difference in identification performance between flanked and single letters) and reading performance for the dyslexic participants revealed that the flanking effect expressed in either RTs or error scores was marginally significantly correlated with performance in the word-reading task [$r = -.34$, $p = .054$, one-tailed, for RTs; $r = -.31$, $p = .07$, one-tailed, for error scores]. If the RTs and the error scores were both converted to z scores and subsequently averaged for each participant (in order to account for a possible speed-accuracy trade-off in the flanking effect), the correlation was significant [$r = -.38$, $p < .05$, one-tailed]. As can be seen in Figure 5a, the dyslexic participants who had the largest problems with the flankers were (on the average) those that read the smallest number of words in the word-reading task. (For the nonwords, the correlations were in the same direction but they were non-significant. As to the normal readers, reading performance was far less variable than for the dyslexic readers and was near ceiling. No significant correlations were found for these readers.) Further, in an unpublished follow-up study (Omtzigt and Hendriks), with a group of 24 normally reading university students performing essentially the same sequence of tasks as in the present study, a significant correlation was obtained between the flanking effect and performance in the nonword-reading task [$r = -.13$, *ns*, for RTs; $r = -.51$, $p < .01$, one-tailed, for error scores; $r = -.36$, $p < .05$, one-tailed, for averaged z scores], which had been adapted so as to avoid ceiling effects (the adjustment proved insufficient to prevent ceiling effects in the word-reading task, however) (see Figure 5b).

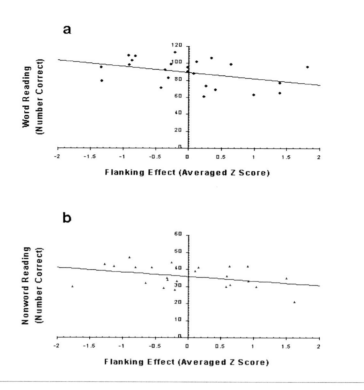

Figure 5. Scatter diagram for: (a) performance in the word-reading task (number correct) by flanking effect (averaged z score) for the dyslexic readers in the present study; (b) performance in the nonword-reading task (number correct) by flanking effect (averaged z score) for the normal readers in Omtzigt and Hendriks (unpublished results).

A contrast manipulation such as used in the present study has the desirable property that it makes possible an investigation of magnocellular-input-dependent mechanisms in reading in a relatively simple and direct way. It has already yielded that magnocellular input is important to the identification of flanked letters (Omtzigt et al., 2002), and a recent study has suggested that this is due to involvement of magnocellular input in the directing of attention onto the target letter (Omtzigt and Hendriks, 2004). If a magnocellular deficit is indeed the cause of poor flanked-letter identification in developmental dyslexia, a follow-up study taking care of the points noted may well provide the definitive test.

AUTHOR NOTE

This study was conducted in partial fulfilment of the requirements for the degree of Doctor of Social Sciences at Radboud University Nijmegen (first author). The authors wish to thank Marij de Rooij from Dienst Studentenzaken at Radboud University Nijmegen for her co-operation in recruiting dyslexic participants, Anna Bosman for the idea of and Debby Wilschut for the clear articulation in the phonological nonword-reversal task, Hubert Voogd for the provision of computer-programming assistance, and Eric Maris for statistical advice.

REFERENCES

Amitay, S., Ben-Yehudah, G., Banai, K., and Ahissar, M. (2002). Disabled readers suffer from visual and auditory impairments but not from a specific magnocellular deficit. *Brain,* 125, 2272-2285.

Atkinson, J. (1991). Review of human visual development: crowding and dyslexia. In J. F. Stein (Ed.), *Vision and visual dyslexia* (pp. 44-57). Houndmills, UK: MacMillan Press.

Atkinson, J. (1993). Vision in dyslexics: letter recognition acuity, visual crowding, contrast sensitivity, accommodation, convergence and sight reading music. In S. F. Wright and R. Groner (Eds.), *Facets of dyslexia and its remediation* (pp. 125-138). Amsterdam: Elsevier Science Publishers.

Boder, E. (1973). Developmental dyslexia: a diagnostic approach based on three atypical reading-spelling patterns. *Developmental Medicine and Child Neurology,* 15, 663-687.

Borsting, E., Ridder III, W. H., Dudeck, K., Kelly, C., Matsui, L., and Motoyama, J. (1996). The presence of a magnocellular defect depends on the type of dyslexia. *Vision Research,* 36, 1047-1053.

Bouma, H., and Legein, C. P. (1977). Foveal and parafoveal recognition of letters and words by dyslexics and by average readers. *Neuropsychologia,* 15, 69-80.

Bouma, H., and Legein, C. P. (1980). Dyslexia: a specific recoding deficit? An analysis of response latencies for letters and words in dyslectics and in average readers. *Neuropsychologia,* 18, 285-298.

Brus, B. T., and Voeten, M. J. M. (1999). *Een-Minuut-Test.* Lisse, the Netherlands: Swets and Zeitlinger.

Cestnick, L., and Coltheart, M. (1999). The relationship between language-processing and visual-processing deficits in developmental dyslexia. *Cognition,* 71, 231-255.

Chase, C., Ashourzadeh, A., Kelly, C., Monfette, S., and Kinsey, K. (2003). Can the magnocellular pathway read? Evidence from studies of color. *Vision Research,* 43, 1211-1222.

Cornelissen, P. L., Hansen, P. C., Hutton, J. L., Evangelinou, V., and Stein, J. F. (1998). Magnocellular visual function and children's single word reading. *Vision Research,* 38, 471-482.

Cornelissen, P., Richardson, A., Mason, A., Fowler, S., and Stein, J. (1995). Contrast sensitivity and coherent motion detection measured at photopic luminance levels in dyslexics and controls. *Vision Research,* 35, 1483-1494.

Demb, J. B., Boynton, G. M., Best, M., and Heeger, D. J. (1998). Psychophysical evidence for a magnocellular pathway deficit in dyslexia. *Vision Research,* 38, 1555-1559.

Deubel, H., and Schneider, W. X. (1996). Saccade target selection and object recognition: evidence for a common attentional mechanism. *Vision Research,* 36, 1827-1837.

Eden, G. F., VanMeter, J. W., Rumsey, J. M., Maisog, J. M., Woods, R. P., and Zeffiro, T. A. (1996). Abnormal processing of visual motion in dyslexia revealed by functional brain imaging. *Nature,* 382, 66-69.

Eriksen, B. A., and Eriksen, C. W. (1974). Effects of noise letters upon the identification of a target letter in a nonsearch task. *Perception and Psychophysics,* 16, 143-149.

Facoetti, A. (2001). Facilitation and inhibition mechanisms of human visuospatial attention in a non-search task. *Neuroscience Letters,* 298, 45-48.

Facoetti, A., Lorusso, M. L., Paganoni, P., Cattaneo, C., Galli, R., and Mascetti, G. G. (2003). The time course of attentional focusing in dyslexic and normally reading children. *Brain and Cognition,* 53, 181-184.

Facoetti, A., Paganoni, P., Turatto, M., Marzola, V. and Mascetti, G. G. (2000). Visual-spatial attention in developmental dyslexia. *Cortex,* 36, 109-123.

Facoetti, A., and Turatto, M. (2000). Asymmetrical visual fields distribution of attention in dyslexic children: a neuropsychological study. *Neuroscience Letters,* 290, 216-218.

Farrag, A. F., Khedr, E. M., and Abel-Naser, W. (2002). Impaired parvocellular pathway in dyslexic children. *European Journal of Neurology,* 9, 359-363.

Habib, M. (2000). The neurological basis of developmental dyslexia. An overview and working hypothesis. *Brain,* 123, 2373-2399.

Hansen, P. C., Stein, J. F., Orde, S. R., Winter, J. L., and Talcott, J. B. (2001). Are dyslexics' visual deficits limited to measures of dorsal stream function? *NeuroReport,* 12, 1527-1530.

Hari, R., and Renvall, H. (2001). Impaired processing of rapid stimulus sequences in dyslexia. *Trends in Cognitive Sciences,* 5, 525-532.

Hari, R., and Renvall, H., and Tanskanen, T. (2001). Left minineglect in dyslexic adults. *Brain,* 124, 1373-1380.

Hill, G. T., and Raymond, J. E. (2002). Deficits of motion transparency perception in adult developmental dyslexics with normal unidirectional motion sensitivity. *Vision Research,* 42, 1195-1203.

Huckauf, A., and Heller, D. (2002). Spatial selection in peripheral letter recognition: in search of boundary conditions. *Acta Psychologica,* 111, 101-123.

Intriligator, J., and Cavanagh, P. (2001). The spatial resolution of visual attention. *Cognitive Psychology,* 43, 171-216.

Klein, R. M., and D'Entremont, B. (1999). Filtering performance by good and poor readers. In: J. Everatt (Ed.), *Reading and dyslexia: visual and attentional processes* (pp. 163-178). London: Routledge.

Leat, S. J., Li, W., and Epp, K. (1999). Crowding in central and eccentric vision: the effects of contour interaction and attention. *Investigative Ophthalmology and Visual Science,* 40, 504-512.

Ley, R. (1979). F curves have two tails but the F test is a one-tailed two-tailed test. *Journal of Behavior Therapy and Experimental Psychiatry,* 10, 207-212.

Livingstone, M., and Hubel, D. (1988). Segregation of form, color, movement, and depth: anatomy, physiology, and perception. *Science,* 240, 740-749.

Livingstone, M. S., Rosen, G. D., Drislane, F. W., and Galaburda, A. M. (1991). Physiological and anatomical evidence for a magnocellular defect in developmental dyslexia. *Proceedings of the National Academy of Sciences of the United States of America,* 88, 7943-7947.

Luteijn, F., and Van der Ploeg, F. A. E. (1983). *Groninger Intelligentie Test (GIT).* Lisse, the Netherlands: Swets and Zeitlinger.

Maunsell, J. H. R. (1992). Functional visual streams. *Current Opinion in Neurobiology,* 2, 506-510.

McPeek, R. M., Maljkovic, V., and Nakayama, K. (1999). Saccades require focal attention and are facilitated by a short-term memory system. *Vision Research,* 39, 1555-1566.

Milner, A. D., and Goodale, M. A. (1995). *The visual brain in action.* New York: Oxford University Press.

O'Brien, B. A. (1997). Luminance and chromatic contrast effects on skilled and disabled reading performed with and without required eye movements (Doctoral dissertation, Tulane University, 1996). *Dissertation Abstracts International B,* 57, 4756.

Omtzigt, D., and Hendriks, A. W. (2004). Magnocellular involvement in flanked-letter identification relates to the allocation of attention. *Vision Research,* 44, 1927-1940.

Omtzigt, D., Hendriks, A. W., and Kolk, H. H. J. (2002). Evidence for magnocellular involvement in the identification of flanked letters. *Neuropsychologia,* 40, 1881-1890.

Orton, S. T. (1937). *Reading, writing and speech problems in children.* New York: W. W. Norton and Company, Inc.

Pammer, K., and Wheatley, C. (2001). Isolating the M(y)-cell response in dyslexia using the spatial frequency doubling illusion. *Vision Research,* 41, 2139-2147.

Ramus, F., Rosen, S., Dakin, S. C., Day, B. L., Castellote, J. M., White, S., and Frith, U. (2003). Theories of developmental dyslexia: insights from a multiple case study of dyslexic adults. *Brain,* 126, 841-865.

Raymond, J. E. (2000). Attentional modulation of visual motion perception. *Trends in Cognitive Sciences,* 4, 42-50.

Raymond, J. E., and Sorensen, R. E. (1998). Visual motion perception in children with dyslexia: normal detection but abnormal integration. *Visual Cognition,* 5, 389-404.

Rayner, K. (1998). Eye movements in reading and information processing: 20 years of research. *Psychological Bulletin,* 124, 372-422.

Ridder III, W. H., Borsting, E., and Banton, T. (2001). All developmental dyslexic subtypes display an elevated motion coherence threshold. *Optometry and Vision Science,* 78, 510-517.

Ridder III, W. H., Borsting, E., Cooper, M., McNeel, B., and Huang, E. (1997). Not all dyslexics are created equal. *Optometry and Vision Science,* 74, 99-104.

Shepherd, M., Findlay, J. M., and Hockey, R. J. (1986). The relationship between eye movements and spatial attention. *Quarterly Journal of Experimental Psychology,* 38A, 475-491.

Shiu, L.-P., and Pashler, H. (1995). Spatial attention and Vernier acuity. *Vision Research,* 35, 337-343.

Skottun, B. C. (2000). The magnocellular deficit theory of dyslexia: the evidence from contrast sensitivity. *Vision Research,* 40, 111-127.

Slaghuis, W. L., and Lovegrove, W. J. (1985). Spatial-frequency-dependent visible persistence and specific reading disability. *Brain and Cognition,* 4, 219-240.

Slaghuis, W. L., and Ryan, J. F. (1999). Spatio-temporal contrast sensitivity, coherent motion, and visible persistence in developmental dyslexia. *Vision Research, 39*, 651-668.

Snowling, M. J. (2000). *Dyslexia* (2nd ed.). Oxford, UK: Blackwell Publishers.

Spinelli, D., De Luca, M., Judica, A., and Zoccolotti, P. (2002). Crowding effects on word identification in developmental dyslexia. *Cortex, 38*, 179-200.

Stein, J. (2003). Visual motion sensitivity and reading. *Neuropsychologia, 41*, 1785-1793.

Stein, J., and Walsh, V. (1997). To see but not to read; the magnocellular theory of dyslexia. *Trends in Neurosciences, 20*, 147-152.

Steinman, S. B., Steinman, B. A., and Garzia, R. (1998). Vision and attention. II: Is visual attention a mechanism through which a deficient magnocellular pathway might cause reading disability? *Optometry and Vision Science, 75*, 674-681.

Strasburger, H., Harvey Jr., L. O., and Rentschler, I. (1991). Contrast thresholds for identification of numeric characters in direct and eccentric view. *Perception and Psychophysics, 49*, 495-508.

Stuart, G. W., McAnally, K. I., and Castles, A. (2001). Can contrast sensitivity functions in dyslexia be explained by inattention rather than a magnocellular deficit? *Vision Research, 41*, 3205-3211.

Talcott, J. B., Hansen, P. C., Assoku, E. L., and Stein, J. F. (2000). Visual motion sensitivity in dyslexia: evidence for temporal and energy integration deficits. *Neuropsychologia, 38*, 935-943.

Ungerleider, L. G., and Haxby, J. V. (1994). "What" and "where" in the human brain. *Current Opinion in Neurobiology, 4*, 157-165.

Van den Bos, K. P., Lutje Spelberg, H. C., Scheepsma, A. J. M., and De Vries, J. R. (1999). *De Klepel.* Lisse, the Netherlands: Swets and Zeitlinger.

Vidyasagar, T. R. (1999). A neuronal model of attentional spotlight: parietal guiding the temporal. *Brain Research Reviews, 30*, 66-76.

Vidyasagar, T. R., and Pammer, K. (1999). Impaired visual search in dyslexia relates to the role of the magnocellular pathway in attention. *NeuroReport, 10*, 1283-1287.

Witton, C., Talcott, J. B., Hansen, P. C., Richardson, A. J., Griffiths, T. D., Rees, A., Stein, J. F., and Green, G. G. R. (1998). Sensitivity to dynamic auditory and visual stimuli predicts nonword reading ability in both dyslexic and normal readers. *Current Biology, 8*, 791-797.

Wolford, G., and Chambers, L. (1983). Lateral masking as a function of spacing. *Perception and Psychophysics, 33*, 129-138.

In: Dyslexia in Children: New Research
Editor: Christopher B. Hayes, pp. 143-160

ISBN 1-59454-969-9
© 2006 Nova Science Publishers, Inc.

Chapter 8

TRAINING VISUAL-SPATIAL ATTENTION IN DEVELOPMENTAL DYSLEXIA

Maria Luisa Lorusso[1], Andrea Facoetti[1,2], Carmen Cattaneo[1], Silvia Pesenti[1], Raffaella Galli[1], Massimo Molteni[1] and Gad Geiger[3]

[1] Scientific Institute "E. Medea", Bosisio Parini, Italy
[2] Dept. of General Psychology, University of Padua, Italy
[3] Center for Biological and Computational Learning and the McGovern Institute
for Brain Research – Brain and Cognitive Sciences,
Massachusetts Institute of Technology, Cambridge, MA

ABSTRACT

Recent studies have shown the critical role of the ability to actively select visual information (attentional focusing) in developmental dyslexia. A program specifically devised by Geiger and Lettvin to train selection of visual information and small-scale focusing has been tried out with a group of 16 dyslexic children. The results after a three-months training have been compared with those obtained by another group of 11 dyslexic children after the same period of customary reading training in a speech-therapy context. All children were assessed on reading, spelling and phonemic awareness and their FRFs (Form-Resolving Fields), i.e. the extent of their field of correct visual recognition, were measured. The children who followed the experimental training improved their reading and spelling performances as much as the children who were treated by speech therapists (no significant differences were observed between the two groups). However, separate analyses reveal that improvements after treatment for the experimental group on reading accuracy, reading speed, spelling, phonemic awareness reached statistical significance. The group receiving customary speech therapy, on the other hand, shows significant improvements on spelling only.

Keywords: developmental dyslexia, intervention, lateral masking, peripheral vision, visual attention.

INTRODUCTION

A wide variety of treatment approaches for developmental dyslexia have been attempted with children in the past (e.g., Bradley and Bryant, 1983; Snowling, 1987). However, very few have been theoretically based, controlled intervention studies, so that little information is available concerning treatment efficacy (Brunsdon, Hannan, Nickels,and Coltheart, 2002; Eden and Moats, 2002).

Most of these remediation programs, indeed, are based on training of phonological and metaphonological skills. In the last few decades, in fact, research on developmental dyslexia has pointed to phonological deficits as the main cause of reading difficulties (Bradley and Bryant, 1983; Liberman, Shankweiler, Fischer, and Carter 1974, Snowling, 2001). Moreover, the few controlled studies on the effectiveness of remediation programs based on visual-perceptual abilities or on visual-motor skills had proven greatly disappointing, both in terms of their effects on reading abilities, and in terms of their effects on perceptual-motor performance itself (Hammill, Goodman and Wiederholt, 1974; Wise and Olson, 1991).

In recent years, however, renewed interest has been devoted to the visual aspects of reading and dyslexia, especially reformulated in terms of the "Magnocellular theory of dyslexia" (Stein and Walsh, 1997), or pointing to specific visual-perceptual or visual-attentional processes (Casco, Tressoldi and Dellantonio, 1998; Cestnick and Coltheart, 1999; Hari and Renvall, 2001; Facoetti and Molteni, 2001; Facoetti, Paganoni and Lorusso, 2000).

Lovegrove and MacFarlane (1990), and Hill and Lovegrove (1993) showed that reading difficulties are more evident when an individual is asked to read words embedded in text than single words. This may be interpreted as a lack of coordination between peripheral and foveal vision, and may be related to the phenomenon of lateral masking, which is suggested to account for the dyslexics' greater difficulties at reading strings of letters than single letters (Bouma and Legein, 1977).

Lateral masking, which is sometimes referred to as "visual crowding" (Atkinson, 1991), is the process by which a visual stimulus becomes less recognizable when flanked by other visual elements. If lateral masking in the periphery is not effective, visual information from the entire surroundings is simultaneously perceived, which may result in confusion (Geiger et al., 1992).

In order to measure the spatial distribution of lateral masking, Geiger and colleagues designed a letter recognition task where pairs of letters are presented briefly, one at the centre of gaze and one in the periphery (along the horizontal axis). The plot of the recognition rate of the peripheral letter against eccentricity was named FRF (Form Resolving Field) by Geiger and coll.. While the FRF of ordinary readers is reasonably symmetrical, its shape in adult dyslexic readers is significantly wider in the direction of reading (Geiger et al., 1992; Perry, Dember, Warm, and Sacks, 1989; Dautrich, 1993). Moreover, while ordinary readers recognize the peripheral letters best when they are nearest to the centre of gaze, for dyslexic readers best recognition on the right is at some distance from the fixation point. In dyslexic children, the distribution of lateral masking is as wide as, but less asymmetric than in adults (Geiger et al.,1994). The ratio of recognition in the centre and in the periphery of the visual field is captured by a numerical index, called Criterion 2 (CR2), that was found to accurately discriminate dyslexic from ordinary readers (Lorusso, Facoetti, Pesenti, Cattaneo, Molteni, and Geiger, 2004).

Geiger and Lettvin (1987, 1999) proposed that the process of lateral masking is active, and its distribution is learned with practice and is task-dependent. On the basis of these observations, they devised a training program specifically aiming at changing dyslexic individuals' visual strategies in order to facilitate reading processes.

Geiger, Lettvin and Zegarra-Moran (1992) first demonstrated that dyslexics' visual strategies can be changed. The case is presented of four severe dyslexics who were subjected to a training practice consisting of two separate, complementary parts. The first part required them to devote two hours every day to novel, small-scale, hand-eye coordination tasks such as drawing, model-building etc.. The second part consisted in trying to read through a "window" in the peripheral field. A blank sheet was laid over the text to be read, with a rectangular cut (the "window") as long as an average word, and a mark drawn to the left of the window, representing the fixation point. The distance from the fixation point to the center of the window was set by using the eccentricity of the peak of the individual FRF (i.e. the point at which lateral masking was least effective in masking the peripheral letter). The subjects had to gaze on the fixation point and read what appeared in the window, then shift the sheet to read the next word on the right, and so on. After about four months of practice, the subjects were tested again. Their reading (comprehension, word recognition, reading and writing) performance improved consistently, and their FRFs dramatically changed so as to become indistinguishable from those of ordinary readers.

In Geiger, Lettvin and Fahle's study (1994) nine dyslexic children from 3rd to 6th grade were subjected to the same regimen of novel small-scale hand-eye coordination tasks and reading word-by-word trough a "window". The children practiced for at least half an hour daily each of the two regimen components. A control group (six children) continued their remedial procedure at school. After three months, all children were re-tested. The children who had practiced with the experimental program increased their reading abilities by 1,22 grade-levels on average, while the children in the control group showed only minimal (and significantly less) improvement. In the meantime, the FRF of the experimental group narrowed significantly on the right side but not on the left side, while no change was observed in the control group. In an extended study using the same paradigm with a larger group of children (49), Fahle and Luberichs (1995) found significant improvement (although less evident than the previous study) after two-three months of practice with the Geiger-Lettvin method, both in reading and in spelling. The children's FRFs, however, did not show any significant changes. As a conclusion, Fahle and Luberichs suggested that the effectiveness of the method, though generally positive, may be influenced by subjects' characteristics such as age and initial reading level, the children included in their study being older (9-13 y.o.) and less severely impaired in reading than the children in Geiger et al.'s (1994) study. On the basis of anecdotic evidence, Geiger and Lettvin (2000) also suggest that practicing only one of the two parts of the regimen does not produce comparable improvements in reading. Only the combined effects of better attentional focusing (by means of hand-eye coordination practice) and better word identification abilities resulted in improvement of reading abilities. In a recent study, Geiger and Amara (2005) showed that one year-long extensive practice of hand-eye coordination activities in a group of kindergarten, first and second grade children significantly reduced the number of children at-risk for reading problems (11.76%, compared with 24,69% in the control group).

It can be concluded that the results of the practice regimen suggested by Geiger and Lettvin have so far been encouraging. Although slightly different in their practical procedures, the same principles have also been applied in designing other forms of remedial training for dyslexia. Iozzino, Montanari and Palla (reported in Tressoldi, Vio, Lorusso, Facoetti, and Iozzino, 2003) had a group of dyslexic children treated with a program consisting of reading text masked on the right side and single words masked on the left and the right side, for about 10 min. per day, and a total duration of about three months. The children improved their reading speed of .40 syll/sec and their mean error score in text reading decreased of 7 units (errors).

The present study aims at testing the effectiveness of Geiger and Lettvin's practice program in a group of Italian dyslexic children, recruited in a clinical setting, working at their homes, and comparing it with a traditional intervention program, carried out by speech therapists in a clinical framework.

METHODS

Participants

At the beginning of the study, 42 dyslexic children, native Italian speakers, aged between 7 and 15 years, were included in the study.

The children had been referred to the Unit of Cognitive Psychology and Neuropsychology of Scientific Institute "E. Medea", or to the corresponding units of the collaborating centres, because of learning difficulties. Assessment and diagnosis were performed at either Scientific Institute "E. Medea" or at Bergamo Hospital. The diagnosis of developmental dyslexia was made according to ICD-10 criteria (1992): Full-scale IQ (as assessed by the Wechsler Intelligence Scale for Children-Revised, Italian version - Wechsler, 1986) equal to, or higher than, 85; at least 1 SD below age mean of either accuracy or speed scores in reading a text aloud; at least one score below 2 SDs on any of the reading and spelling tests which were included in the psychometric testing. Moreover, they had no reports of neurological or psychiatric problems, or major emotional and social problems. Their language comprehension, assessed through the abridged version of the Token Test (Di Simoni, 1978) was not inferior to 2 SD with respect to age norms. Children who scored under 2 SDs in spelling tests alone were included only if they had a documented history of preceding reading problems (ICD-10, 1992).

All the children had normal or trivially corrected-to-normal vision.

Thirty children received Visual Spatial Attention Training (VSAT group), while the remaining eleven children underwent traditional Speech Therapy (ST group). Assignment of the dyslexic children to the two groups was decided according to the distance from the children's homes to the Institute, so that children who lived far were given the possibility to follow a rehabilitation program at home. After four months, average time spent daily on each part of the VSAT practice (see Methods section) was calculated for each child included in the VSAT group. Only sixteen of the children reached the minimum average of time (at least 10 min.) spent on each of the two parts of the regimen and were accepted for final inclusion in the experimental sample.

The distribution of demographic and socio-economic variables, as well as the proportion of children who lived in cities and in rural areas, were comparable in the two groups. A comparable distribution of cases with respect to sex, IQ, age and dyslexia subtype was also ensured. A Fisher's Exact test revealed no significant differences in the distribution of dyslexia subtypes in the two groups, classified as P-, L- or M-types according to Bakker (1990) ($P > .05$). Further, the two groups did not differ in pre-treatment reading and spelling performances (all $Ps > .5$).

Descriptive data of the children in the two groups are reported in Table 1.

Table 1. Descriptive data of the two groups

	VSAT	Speech Therapy
Number and sex of participants	16 (13 males and 3 females)	11 (7 males and 4 females)
Mean age (DS)	10.24 (2.31)	10.92 (1.95)
Mean full IQ (DS)	105.20 (16.44)	96.64 (5.91)
P-types	7	2
L-types	2	1
M-types	7	8

Data from the group of children who had first been assigned to the VSAT group but had practiced for less than the minimum average time were also analyzed and considered as a further, "no-treatment" control group.

Testing Procedures

All children were tested before and after treatment. Assessment involved reading and spelling skills, metaphonologic skills and FRF. Tests commonly used in the assessment of reading disabilities in Italy were used. All of the tests have age norms and satisfactory validity and reliability scores.

The results of the tests, with the exception of the metaphonological tasks, are expressed as z-scores according to age norms.

The following tests were administered in the pre- and post-test sessions:

1) *Text Reading*: "Prove di rapidità e correttezza nella lettura del gruppo MT" ("Test for speed and accuracy in reading, developed by the MT group") (Cornoldi, Colpo, and Gruppo MT, 1986), a text-reading task meant to assess reading abilities for meaningful material. It provides separate scores for speed and accuracy. Texts increase in complexity with grade level. Norms are provided for each text. This task was also used for classification of dyslexia according to Bakker's model (P-, L-, M-type), based on error type and reading times (see Bakker, 1979, 1990).

2) *Single word/non-word reading:* "Batteria per la Valutazione della Dislessia e Disortografia Evolutiva" (Battery for the assessment of Developmental Reading and Spelling Disorders), (Sartori, Job, and Tressoldi, 1995).

This test assesses speed and accuracy (expressed in number of errors) in reading word lists (4 lists of 24 words) and non-word lists (3 lists of 16 non-words) and provides grade norms from the second to the last grade of junior high school.

3) *Spelling tests:* "Batteria per la Valutazione della Dislessia e Disortografia Evolutiva" (Battery for the assessment of Developmental Reading and Spelling Disorders), (Sartori et al., 1995). The battery includes three dictation tasks, giving correctness scores in writing words (48), non-words (24) and sentences (12) for children/adolescents from the second grade to the last grade of junior high school.

4) *Tests of phonemic awareness* (Cossu, Shankweiler, Liberman, Katz, and Tola, 1988).

- phonemic elision: the test assesses the ability to recognize and isolate the phonemic constituents of 20 words (in this specific case, the initial constituents). The child is asked to delete the first two phonemes in the word read by the examiner and to report the resulting non-word.
- phoneme synthesis: this task assesses the capacity to derive a phonemic pattern from distinct phonemic units. The examiner presents each of 20 words letter by letter and the child is requested to identify and report the resulting word.

For both tasks, the scores refer to the total number of errors. Only age means (as raw scores) are provided.

Procedure for FRF Measurement

The procedure was the same as in Lorusso et al. (2004). The subjects were asked to gaze at the fixation point on a milk-glass screen. After a verbal warning, a slide was projected replacing the fixation point. The slide showed two letters, one in the center (at fixation point) and one at varying eccentricities to the right or to the left of fixation point. The subject was requested to name the two letters and specify their positions. Stimulus duration was determined individually for each subject (after Geiger et al., 1992) and kept for the entire measurement. It ranged between 3 and 60 msec. Individual average presentation time is referred to as Teff (effective duration). After presenting all the stimuli, a plot of correct identification of the peripheral letter, as a function of eccentricity, was made. This plot represents the FRF. The score of correct identification of the central letters was given numerically. To characterize the width of each FRF, the ratio between the recognition rate at 2.5 deg and the sum of the recognition rates at 10 and 12.5 deg eccentricity was calculated. Since the shape of the FRF for dyslexics is wider to the right, which is the reading direction of English and Italian, this side only was considered. We refer to this ratio as to "Criterion 2" (CR2).

That is:

$$CR2 = \frac{\%correct,\,at\,2.5\,deg.}{\%correct,\,at\,10\,deg. + \%correct,\,at\,12.5\,deg.}$$

Children whose CR2 was greater than 2 were considered as normal readers; children whose CR2 was equal to, or less than, 2, were considered as dyslexic readers.

Treatment

Both treatment programs were carried out over a 4 months' period. Parents and teachers of the children who took part in the study were contacted to ensure that no other specific activity for remediation of the reading difficulty was conducted during the study.

1) Geiger and Lettvin's Visual-Spatial Attention training (VSAT)

The VSAT consists of two main parts:

a) hand-eye coordination tasks, that have to be carried out by the child for about one hour daily. The main feature of the tasks is that their execution requires a very precise perceptual analysis and monitoring of the task and the material. In particular, the task should require visual attention to be focussed on a very limited part of the visual space. In order to avoid automatic (and therefore less controlled and less focussed) processing of the task, it should be new and unfamiliar to the child. Moreover, the task should be motivating for the child, and possibly be conceived as a game or a hobby, rather than as an exercise. For these reasons, a list of wide-ranging types of activities was given to the children, but they were free to choose the tasks that they found most interesting, and to add any other activity, provided that it respected the essential features of the training (small pieces to be handled, precision work). The list included drawing and painting, various techniques for art-work, knitting, sawing, making puppets, mechanical or electric constructions, and further, games as origami, Lego, Shanghai, Spirograph etc.

b) reading text through a rectangular cut (window) in a blank sheet (frame). A dot was marked on the frame, left of the window, to indicate fixation point during reading. The distance of the fixation point from the window was determined according to the point of best recognition in the FRF. The size of the window was such that about a single word, or parts of long words, could be read at a time. The children were asked to read through the window, with the frame laid on the text, for at least half an hour daily. They were free to decide if they preferred to read silently or aloud. The children were also allowed to take the frame with them and use it at school, if they liked to.

The training could be carried out at the children's homes, and the child received all the instructions that enabled him/her to organize his/her own activities without the need of a strict supervision by parents. A psychologist was in charge of keeping the contacts with each family through monthly phone-calls. In each phone-call, the child was interviewed about the work he/she had been doing in the month, whether he/she had enjoyed it, and if he/she had the feeling that it was useful. Suggestions and encouragement were given to the child as to the prosecution of the work. The parents were also asked to report the average daily amount of work that their child was doing. The average time spent training each part of the program was recorded as reported by the child and his /her parents (in case of discordant data, a further enquiry was made in order to estimate the actual amount and duration of work).

2) Speech therapy (ST)

Treatment took place at the outpatient clinic of the rehabilitation institute "E. Medea" and at the Neuropsychiatric Unit of Bergamo Hospital, and was carried out by trained speech therapists. The term "traditional ST" refers to the kind of intervention that is commonly adopted by speech therapists to treat specific reading disorders. It can be considered to be the "default" treatment of dyslexia in most Italian public health services. The treatment is based on various existing intervention programs for remediation of dyslexia. Specific tasks focus mainly on some reading sub-processes (phonological, perceptual pre-requisites), re-education using guided reading tasks, or strengthening of compensatory strategies. The range of activities that the children would be involved with had been discussed within the whole group of therapists before the beginning of the study. The therapists agreed upon a common general protocol, but they were entitled to choose among the various tasks the ones that they considered to be most appropriate for each child, according to age and functional profile. On the whole, the individual programs, although not identical, could be considered as homogeneous enough to be treated as one single group.

RESULTS

Pre and Post-Treatment Assessment

Effectiveness of both methods was assessed by comparing performance on the various tests before and after treatment. Raw scores (with the exception of phonemic- awareness scores) were transformed into z-scores, according to age norms.

Four global scores were computed:

a) *global accuracy score*, i.e. the average of accuracy scores in text, word and non-word reading
b) *global speed score*, i.e. the average of speed scores in text, word and non-word reading
c) *global spelling score*, i.e. the average of scores in word, non-word and sentence writing from dictation
d) *global phonemic awareness error score*, i.e. the average of phonemic synthesis and phonemic elision error scores

First of all, a comparison of the initial performances by the two groups on these global scores confirmed the absence of significant differences on any of the scores (all p-values ≥ .5).

CR2 were computed from individual FRFs and group averages were calculated. Mean CR2 and Teff in the two groups, together with medians and ranges, are presented in Table 2. As expected, the mean and median values of CR2 are in the "dyslexic" range, i.e. below 2. Specifically, for 25 out of 27 children (92%), CR2 was congruent with the diagnosis based on clinical assessment. This is in line with previous findings (Lorusso et al., 2004). No differences were found in CR2 between different dyslexia subtypes according to Bakker's typology (p = .99).

**Table 2. Mean values and distribution of CR2 and
Teff, in the two groups (VSAT and ST)**

		mean	median	sd	max	min
VSAT group	CR2	1,51	1,43	0,75	4,00	0,83
	Teff [ms]	12,25	9,00	5,87	28,5	7,5
ST group	CR2	1,68	1,67	0,64	3,30	1,00
	Teff [ms]	9,67	9,50	2,48	14,5	6,5

An analysis of variance (ANOVA) with Group (VSAT vs ST) as a between-subjects factor and Time (pre-test vs post-test) as a within-subjects factor was performed on all global scores (see Table 3). A significant main effect of Time emerged, to indicate significant improvement in all children after treatment, while the effects of Group and Group-by-Time interaction were not significant.

**Table 3. Significance levels of the main effects (time and group) and group x time
interactions on the global scores (repeated measures ANOVA)**

TASKS	Time effect (before vs after)	Group effect (VSAT vs ST)	Group x Time interaction (improvement in VSAT vs ST)
Global accuracy score	$F (25,1) = 12.62$ $P = .002$	ns	ns
Global speed score	$F (25,1) = 7.12$ $P = .013$	ns	ns
Global writing score	$F (23,1) = 15.79$ $P = .001$	ns	ns
Global phonemic awareness score	$F (24,1) = 13.83$ $P = .001$	ns	ns

In order to look for more subtle differences between the two groups, a t-test was subsequently performed on each global score, comparing performance before and after treatment for each group, separately. Average scores before and after treatment and the statistical significance of change over time are shown in Table 4, for each group.

The analyses reveal significant improvements after treatment for the VSAT group (see Table 4) on all the global scores: reading accuracy, reading speed, spelling, phonemic awareness. The ST group, on the other hand, shows significant improvements on one global score only, namely spelling.Next, the contribution was investigated of the tests that make up the global scores. A repeated-measures ANOVA was performed with Group as between factor and Test as within factor. In this analysis, the change-scores (i.e. pre-post differences) of the various component tests were compared, to see whether their contribution to improvement in the global score were comparable or not. Neither Test main effects nor Test-by-Group interactions were significant (all Ps > .05). This confirms the validity of the use of global scores in the analyses, and shows that improvement generalized to the various subcomponents of each global score.

Table 4. T-tests comparing pre-treatment and post-treatment global scores,
for each group

TASKS		Before treatment	After treatment	Significance level (1-tailed)	n
VSAT group	Global accuracy score	-2.24 (1.95)	-.76 (1.13)	P < .001	16
	Global speed score	-3.15 (2.42)	-2.12 (2.33)	P < .001	16
	Global spelling score	-2.11 (1.97)	-1.31 (1.73)	P < .05	15
	Global phonemic awareness score	5.28 (3.41)	2.91 (2.64)	P = .001	16
ST group	Global accuracy score	-2.36 (2.54)	-1.67 (2.78)	ns	11
	Global speed score	-2.69 (1.93)	-1.87 (1.1)	ns	11
	Global spelling score	-2.35 (2.18)	-.61 (1.22)	P < .005	10
	Global phonemic awareness score	3.75 (2,79)	2.5 (1.82)	ns	10

As to CR2, describing the FRF, no significant changes were found from pre- to post-test for any of the two groups. However, if two subgroups are considered inside the VSAT group, one above and one below the median of the global accuracy score, it can be observed that a significant change in CR2 is detectable from pre-to post-test (from 1,24 to 1,58 respectively; t (7) = 3.02, p = .02) in the more severely impaired subgroup, while no change at all is present in the less severely impaired subgroup (1.79 and 1.72 pre- and post-test, respectively). This finding supports the hypothesis of a relation between change in the FRF and severity of dyslexia (Fahle and Luberichs, 1995).

Furthermore, change-scores (post-test minus pre-test) were computed for each of the global scores and for CR2. No correlations were found between change in CR2 and change in any of the global scores.

As a final test of the efficacy of the VSAT, a comparison was made on all global scores between the final VSAT sample and the fourteen children who had been excluded because they had practiced for less than 10 min daily on each of the two parts of the program. No significant differences were found in pre-test scores between the two groups (all *ps* > .05). As for change-scores (measuring improvement from pre-to post-test), significant differences were found for the Global Speed score (t (28) = 2.98, *p* = .006) and the Global Phonemic Awareness score (t (28) = 2.24, *p* = .03). Mean average global scores in the two groups before and after treatment, as well as significance levels for improvement, are reported in Table 5. It can be seen that the group who had not practiced for a minimum average time every day (therefore comparable to a no-treatment group, although they did actually do some practice) improved significantly only in one of the four global scores, namely the Global Accuracy score (but less than the VSAT group in absolute amount of improvement).

Table 5. **T-tests comparing pre-treatment and post-treatment global scores, for the group of VSAT children who had not reached the minimum average time spent on training (no-treatment control)**

TASKS		Before treatment	After treatment	Significance level (1-tailed)	n
No-treatment group	Global accuracy score	-2.88 (1.25)	-1.75 (1.43)	P < .005	14
	Global speed score	-4.10 (5.55)	-4.32 (6.28)	ns	14
	Global spelling score	-4.87 (4.55)	-3.74 (4.46)	ns	11
	Global phonemic awareness score	3.96 (2.95)	3.38 (3.59)	ns	13

DISCUSSION

The hypothesis that training visual-spatial attention skills may be beneficial to dyslexic children's reading abilities is supported by the present data. Indeed, the training focused on both fine-scale hand-eye coordination tasks and reading through a window (VSAT) was found to produce at least as much improvement in reading abilities as obtained with a traditional training program focused on reading subskills (ST). While the VSAT group improved significantly in reading speed, reading accuracy, spelling and phonemic awareness, improvement for the children who had undergone ST reached statistical significance on spelling measures only. Moreover, the absence of comparable effects in the group of children who had not reached the minimum average daily time spent on VSAT activities, (except for global correctness, which did show improvement), suggests that improvement cannot be attributed to maturational, educational or aspecific (placebo, Pygmalion effect, etc.) factors.

The effectiveness of VSAT is especially evident for reading skills, while a more moderate trend was found for spelling abilities (specifically, for writing orthographically complex sentences under dictation), which showed slightly greater improvement after ST. This may be an indication that, while reading is more strictly linked to visual-attentional processes, writing (particularly, sentence writing) could be more strongly influenced by metalinguistic abilities that are more directly addressed in a speech-therapy context. However, since the improvement of writing skills was not the main goal in either training method, this result should be considered as secondary. More structured studies, including also other measures of writing abilities would be needed to compare the efficacy of different treatment programs and to understand the meaning of differential effects on spelling performance. Of special interest, on the other hand, is the improvement found in phonemic awareness after VSAT. In fact, children in the VSAT group did not receive any direct training of phonemic awareness skills, while children in the ST group did. It is therefore surprising that VSAT, a training focused on visual-motor skills, produced such striking effects on phonologically-based skills. Of course, it could be argued that increase in phonemic awareness is a result of improved reading skills, or a result of practicing reading through the window. However, the absence of a similar effect in the ST group, that was specifically trained in reading and phonemic skills, as well as in the no-treatment group, who did show improvement in reading accuracy, give little support to this hypothesis. Rather, it seems reasonable to hypothesize that the effects of VSAT were not limited to the visual modality, but encompassed the auditory modality as well. Geiger and Lettvin (2000) already suggested that hand-eye coordination practice and visual recognition of words could influence phonemic awareness skills (although they did not have direct measures of these abilities and their reasoning was based on nonword reading skills), either through the learning of a general, multimodal perceptual strategy, or through the generalization of a visual strategy to the auditory modality. Indeed, recent findings suggest that deficits of selective spatial attention in dyslexia affect more than one sensory modality (Facoetti, Lorusso, Paganoni, Cattaneo, Galli, Umiltà and Mascetti, 2003a; Facoetti, Lorusso, Cattaneo, Galli, and Molteni, 2005), so that it seems plausible to suppose that improvements can also be multimodal.

If one considers that a practice program of the kind suggested by Geiger and Lettvin can be carried out at the children's homes, the present results are of great importance. In fact, they suggest that also children who are not in the position to attend a regular remediation program at a rehabilitation centre or hospital can be offered a possibility to improve their reading abilities without having to leave their homes. Indeed, it should also be observed that of the thirty children who were initially included in the VSAT group, only sixteen were included in the final sample, as the others had not reached the minimum criteria for the amount of practice. Since the children did not differ in their initial reading abilities, it is likely that motivation was what made the difference. This means that only highly motivated children (and supporting families) are likely to be able to keep a constant, sufficient level of activity necessary for improvement to be attained. The absence of direct control on the children's schedules is meant to be an incentive for a sense of responsibility and self-efficacy to be transmitted to the children, yet it can be a disadvantage for the least motivated ones.

From a more speculative point of view, it could be interesting to get more insight in the exact processes that are triggered by VSAT and their relationship with reading abilities. Following Geiger and Lettvin's theory, the training has the aim to change individual visual strategies (taking in as much information as possible from the surrounding) that may be advantageous for some everyday activities, but are ineffective for reading. The theory does not address the question "why" such ineffective strategies are present and persist in dyslexic individuals. Dyslexia is considered as a symptom and addressed as such for remediation. Exploring its remote causes is beyond the scope of the original author's investigations, and beyond the aims (and possibilities) of the present study as well. However, some hypotheses and speculations about the mechanisms that play a role in improving (and possibly in affecting) reading abilities can be put forward.

The change in visual strategies and in the distribution of lateral masking, produced by training and reflected in improvement in reading abilities, has been explained by the Geiger et al. (1992) in the following terms: "Visually guided task performance is based on predicting the content of the next state of perception and having a model of the world (...). An intended next state of perception (...) is achieved efficiently by correcting the error between it and the state predicted from current conditions. (...) In the prediction necessary to perform tasks expertly it is important to single out the relevant from the irrelevant in the welter of information given" (p. 49). Also, "(...) lateral masking is an operation that takes place after perception which is completely sense-driven and before cognition which is apperceptive and arbitrary. Its function is to reduce the informational content communicated by perception" (p. 49). This description entails much of what is usually described as selective attention. The common aspects shared by the mechanism of lateral masking and selective attention can suggest an alternative explanation of the characteristics of visual perception found in dyslexia, in terms of attentional deficits. Despite the great amount of information flooding the natural scenes, we are able to focus attention on one spatial location (and/or object) and to process the relevant information. The major effect on perceptual functions is that focused spatial attention appears to enhance the neural representation of the stimuli. This signal enhancement manifests itself in a variety of ways, including faster reaction times (RTs), improved sensitivity (thresholds), and reduced interactions with flanking stimuli (Facoetti et al., 2005). Focused spatial attention allows decisions to be based on the selected stimulus alone disregarding distracting stimuli (e.g., Braun, 2002; Carrasco and McElree, 2001). "Sluggish attentional shifting" in dyslexic children and adults has been proposed as the cause of their inefficient multi–modal processing of perceptual stimuli (Hari and Renvall, 2001; Facoetti et al., 2003a; Facoetti et al., 2005). Accordingly, several studies have shown deficits in both visual and auditory shifting or focusing of attention in dyslexic subjects. Such a difficulty may be thought to interfere, although in slightly different ways, both with a sequential left-to-right scanning strategy (Cestnick and Coltheart, 1999), and with direct visual recognition of words (Facoetti, Zorzi, Chestnick, Lorusso, Molteni, Paganoni, and Mascetti, in press).

It is more and more widely accepted that visual attention is crucial for perceptual learning (Ahissar and Hochstein, 2002; Vidnyanszky and Sohn, 2005). However, recent psychophysical studies (Green and Bavelier, 2003; Ito, Westheimer, and Gilbert, 1998) have suggested that learning might affect the attentional mechanisms themselves, thus envisaging the possibility of a more crucial role of attention in perceptual learning. Vidnyanszky and Sohn (2005) found that practicing a task that requires selective attention to a specific subset of the visual input results in a more efficient suppression of the processing of simultaneously present task-irrelevant visual stimuli (moving dots). The learning effects (the strength of motion adaptation evoked by the same unattended motion signal) were specific for the direction of the task-irrelevant motion that was present during practice and persisted for several weeks. These results are in agreement with previous studies showing that perceptual learning improves external noise exclusion (Dosher and Lu, 1999; Li, Levi, and Klein, 2004). These studies provide evidence that practice-induced improvement of external noise exclusion is due at least in part to more efficient suppression of the unattended, task-irrelevant visual input. An explanation based on plasticity of attentional selection is also supported by the results of physiological studies which showed that learning affects neural contextual interactions in the visual cortex, including those that mediate attentional modulation (Li, Piech, and Gilbert, 2004).

Other studies have investigated the role of visual attention in the rehabilitation of reading disorders. Facoetti, Lorusso, Paganoni, Umiltà, and Mascetti (2003b) showed that a computerized training program based on Bakker's Balance Model of dyslexia (Bakker, Bouma and Gardien, 1990), employing tachistoscopic presentation of words either in the left or in the right visual field, produces significant improvements not only in reading and spelling abilities (speed and accuracy), but also in attentional focusing as measured by a Posner covert orienting paradigm. In this study, normal readers and dyslexic children differed in their ability to control the visual spatial region of unattended information or to inhibit information in unattended location outside the attentional focus. In fact, normal readers showed the typical RT pattern in covert orienting of attention: a facilitation effect at the attended location caused by the enhancement mechanism and an inhibitory effect at the unattended location caused by a suppression mechanism, both working as integrated processes of selective spatial attention. In contrast, selective spatial attention in dyslexic children seemed to work as a unique enhancement mechanism without the integrated suppression mechanism. After treatment, however, the RT patterns of dyslexic children closely resembled those of normally reading children.

Although we believe that interpretations referring to attentional and perceptual functions are the most adequate and complete to account for all the changes produced by VSAT, it should be acknowledged that other explanations may be proposed.

The first alternative hypothesis certainly concerns the possibility that VSAT stimulates visual and motor functions mediated by the Magnocellular system (Stein and Walsh, 1997), and that reading improvement can thus been explained in this framework. However, the Magnocellular hypothesis fails to explain some of the basic findings of the present line of research on developmental dyslexia, namely the relatively better recognition of letters in the periphery as compared to the centre of the visual field, and therefore this theory does not seem to be most appropriate for interpreting the present data.

Another possible interpretation of the observed effects comes from the studies suggesting that a cerebellar deficit may be the cause of developmental dyslexia. In particular, some authors point to deficits in automatization of reading and of its component functions (such as grapheme-to-phoneme conversion), that they consider to be dependent on deficient cerebellar functioning, as would be suggested by the evidence of poor motor coordination and poor balance in dyslexic children (Nicolson and Fawcett, 1990). Clearly, a practice regimen such as Geiger and Lettvin's one, requiring to improve fine hand-eye and bimanual coordination is very likely to stimulate cerebellar functions, and therefore the cerebellum may be responsible for improvement in reading and spelling abilities. A further, somewhat related explanation concerns the possibility that hand-eye coordination practice improves hemispheric interconncectivity, thus enhancing the efficiency of callosal transfer. Indeed, the hypothesis that dyslexia itself depends on lacking callosal functions has been put forward several times in the literature (Hynd, Obrzut and Bowen, 1987; Gladstone, Best, and Davidson, 1989; Moore, Brown, Markee, Theberge, and Zvi, 1996). In fact, there are some performance similarities between dyslexic individuals and patients with (partial or total) agenesis or disconnection of the corpus callosum, especially in bimanual coordination (Gladstone et al., 1989). Goldberg (1987) proposed a sequence of steps for achieving normal bimanual automaticity that underlines the importance of practice in transferring processing control from premotor systems to subcortical systems (basal ganglia) which gate sensory elements to appropriate prefrontal areas and to the supplementary motor area. According to this author, cerebrocerebellar circuits come later into play to allow more rapid execution. Although both of the last hypotheses provide sensible and important reasons that may explain, at least partly, the effectiveness of VSAT, it could be observed that on might expect dysgraphic problems to benefit in a particular way from this kind of treatment (Mather, 2001), which has not been observed as a core effect in the present and in other studies.

In spite of apparently contradictory and different points of view, all the mentioned explanations are related to a certain extent, and should not be considered as mutually exclusive. Therefore, although the ability to suppress irrelevant information, be it considered as a perceptual or as an attentional process, has been put forward as the main mechanism which is fostered by VSAT and by other similar training programs, it is not unreasonable to suppose that more than one mechanism and more than one function may play a role in producing improvement.

ACKNOWLEDGEMENTS

Special thanks go to the neuropsychiatrists and speech therapists of the Institute "E. Medea" and of Bergamo Hospital for their precious collaboration in the project.

REFERENCES

Ahissar, M., and Hochstein, S. (2002). The role of attention in learning simple visual tasks. In M. Fahle and T. Poggio (Eds.), *Perceptual Learning*. The MIT Press.

Atkinson, J. (1991). Review of human visual development: Crowding and dyslexia. In J. Stein (Ed) *Vision and visual dyslexia*. CRC Press: Boca Raton, pp 44-57.

Bakker, D. J. (1979). Hemispheric differences and reading strategies: Two dyslexias? *Bulletin of the Orton Society, 29,* 84-100.

Bakker, D.J. (1990). *Neuropsychological treatment of dyslexia*. New York: Oxford University Press.

Bakker, D. J., Bouma, A. and Gardien, C. J.(1990). Hemisphere-specific treatment of dyslexia subtypes: A field experiment. *Journal of Learning Disabilities, 23,* 433-438.

Bouma, H. and Legein, Ch.P. (1977). Foveal and parafoveal recognition of letters and words by dyslexic and by average readers. *Neuropsychologia, 15,* 68-80.

Bradley, L. and Bryant, P. (1983). Categorizing sounds and learning to read. A causal connection. *Nature, 301,* 419-421.

Braun, J. (2002). Visual attention: light enters the jungle. *Current Biology,12*, R599-R601.

Brunsdon, R. K., Hannan, T.J., Nickels, L., and Cotheart, M. (2002). Successful treatment of sublexical reading deficits in a child with dyslexia of the mixed type. *Neuropsychological Rehabilitation, 12,* 199-229.

Carrasco, M., and McElree, B. (2001). Covert attention accelerates the rate of visual information processing. *Proceedings of the National Academy of Sciences, 98,* 5363-5367.

Casco, C., Tressoldi, P., and Dellantonio, A. (1998). Visual selective attention and reading efficiency are related in children. *Cortex, 34,* 531-546.

Cestnick, L. and Coltheart, M. (1999). The relationship between language-processing and visual-processing deficits in developmental dyslexia. *Cognition, 71*, 231-255.

Cornoldi, C., Colpo, G., and gruppo MT (1986). *Prove di rapidità e correttezza nella lettura del gruppo MT*. Firenze: Organizzazioni Speciali.

Cossu, G., Shankweiler, D., Liberman, I. Y., Katz, L., and Tola, G. (1988). Awareness of phonological segments and reading ability in Italian children. *Applied Psycholinguistics, 9*, 1-16.

Dautrich, B. (1993). Visual perceptual differences in the dyslexic reader: Evidence of greater visual peripheral sensitivity to color and letter stimuli. *Percept Mot Skills*, 76, 755-764.

Di Simoni, F.G. (1978). *The Token Test for Children*. Allen, TX: DLM Teaching Resources.

Dosher, B., and Lu, Z. (1999). Mechanisms of perceptual learning. *Vision Research, 39*, 3197–3221.

Eden, G. F., and Moats, L. (2002). The role of neuroscience in the remediation of students with dyslexia. *Nature Neuroscience Supplement, 5*, 1080-1084.

Facoetti, A., Lorusso, M. L., Cattaneo, C., Galli, R., and Molteni, M. (2005). Visual and auditory attentional capture are both sluggish in children with developmental dyslexia. *Acta Neurobiologiae Experimentalis, 65*, 61-72.

Facoetti, A., Lorusso, M.L, Paganoni, P., Cattaneo, C., Galli, R., Umiltà, C., and Mascetti, G.G. (2003a). Auditory and visual automatic attention deficits in developmental dyslexia. *Cognitive Brain Research, 16*, 185-191.

Facoetti, A., Lorusso, M.L., Paganoni, P., Umiltà, C., and Mascetti, G.G. (2003b). The role of visuospatial attention in developmental dyslexia: evidence from a rehabilitation study. *Cognitive Brain Research, 15/2*, 154-164.

Facoetti, A., and Molteni, M. (2001). The Gradient Of Visual Attention In Developmental Dyslexia. *Neuropsychologia, 39*, 352-357.

Facoetti, A., Paganoni, M., and Lorusso, M. L. (2000). The spatial distribution of visual attention in developmental dyslexia. *Experimental Brain Research, 132*, 531-538.

Facoetti, A., Zorzi, M., Chestnick, L., Lorusso, M. L., Molteni, M., Paganoni, P., and Mascetti, G. G. (in press). The relationship between visuo-spatial attention and nonword reading in developmental dyslexia. *Cognitive Neuropsychology*.

Fahle, M., and Luberichs, J. (1995). Extension of a recent therapy for dyslexia. *German Journal of Ophtalmology, 4*, 350-354.

Geiger, G., and Amara, D.G. (2005). Towards the prevention of dyslexia. *MIT Computer Science and Artificial Intelligence Laboratory Technical Report, 2005-065*.

Geiger, G. and Lettvin, J.Y. (1987). Peripheral vision in persons with dyslexia. *New England Journal of Medicine, 316*, 1238-1243.

Geiger, G. and Lettvin, J.Y. (1999). How dyslexics see and learn to read well. In J. Everatt (ed.) *Reading and dyslexia: Visual and attentional processes*. London: Routledge, pp.64-90.

Geiger, G. and Lettvin, J.Y. (2000). Developmental dyslexia: a different perceptual strategy and how to learn a new strategy for reading. *Saggi CDandD 26*, 73-89.

Geiger, G. Lettvin, J.Y. and Fahle, M. (1994). Dyslexic Children learn a new visual strategy for reading: a controlled experiment. *Vision Research, 34*, 1223-1233.

Geiger, G., Lettvin, J.Y. and Zegarra-Moran, O. (1992). Task-determined strategies of visual process. *Cognitive Brain Research, 1*, 39-52.

Gladstone, M., Best, C.T., and Davidson, R.J. (1989). Anomalous bimanual coordination among dyslexic boys. *Developmental Psychology, 25*, 236-246.

Goldberg, G. (1987). Premotor systems, motor learning, and ipsilateral control: Learning to get set. *Behavioral and Brain Sciences, 10*, 323-329.

Green, C. S., and Bavelier, D. (2003). Action video game modifies visual selective attention. *Nature, 423*, 534–537.

Hammill, D.D., Goodman, L., and Wiederholt, J.L. (1974). Visual-motor processes: Can we train them? *The Reading Teacher, 27*, 469-478.

Hari, R. and Renvall, H. (2001). Impaired processing of rapid stimulus sequences in dyslexia. *Trends in Cognitive Sciences, 5*, 525-532.

Hill, R. and Lovegrove, W.J. (1993). One word at a time: A solution to the visual deficit in SRDs? In S.F. Groner and R. Groner (eds.) *Facets of dyslexia and its remediation.* North Holland: Elsevier.

Hynd, G. W., Obrzut, J. E., and Bowen, S. M. (1987). Neurological basis of attention and memory in learning disabilities. In H. L. Swanson (Ed.), *Memory and learning disabilities.* Greenwich, CT: JAI Press.

Ito, M., Westheimer, G., and Gilbert, C. D. (1998). Attention and perceptual learning modulate contextual influences on visual perception. *Neuron, 20,* 1191–1197.

Li, R., Levi, D., and Klein, S. (2004). Perceptual learning improves efficiency by re-tuning the decision template for position discrimination. *Nature Neuroscience, 7*, 178–183.

Li, W., Piech, V., and Gilbert, C. D. (2004). Perceptual learning and top–down influences in primary visual cortex. *Nature Neuroscience, 7,*651–657.

Liberman, I., Shankweiler, D., Fischer, F.W. and Carter, B. (1974). Explicit syllable and phoneme segmentation in the young child. *Journal of Experimental Child Psychology*, 18, 201-212.

Lorusso, M.L., Facoetti, A., Pesenti, S., Cattaneo, C., Molteni, M. and Geiger, G. (2004). Wider recognition in peripheral vision for Italian dyslexic children common to different subtypes. *Vision Research, 44,* 2413-2424.

Lovegrove, W. and MacFarlane, T. (1990). The effect of text presentation on reading in dyslexic and normal readers. *Perception, 19*, A46.

Mather, D.S. (2001). Does dyslexia develop from learning the alphabet in the wrong hemisphere? A cognitive neuroscience analysis. *Brain and Language, 76*, 282-316.

Moore, L. H., Brown, W. S., Markee, T. E., Theberge, D. C., and Zvi, J. C. (1996). Callosal transfer of finger localization information in phonologically dyslexic adults. *Cortex, 32*, 311–322.

Nicolson, R.I., and Fawcett, A.J. (1990). Automaticity: a framework for dyslexia research? *Cognition, 35*, 159-182.

Perry, A.R., Dember, W.N., Warm, J.S. and Sacks, J.G. (1989). Letter identification in normal and dyslexic readers: A verification. *Bulletin of the Psychonomic Society, 27,* 445-448.

Sartori, G., Job, R., and Tressoldi, P. E. (1995*). Batteria per la valutazione della dislessia e della disortografia evolutiva.* O.S. Organizzazioni speciali, Firenze.

Snowling, M. (1987). *Dyslexia: A cognitive developmental perspective.* Oxford: Blackwell.

Snowling, M. J. (2001). From language to reading and dyslexia. *Dyslexia, 7*, 37-46.

Stein, J. and Walsh, V. (1997). To see but not to read: The magnocellular theory of dyslexia. *Trends in Neuroscience, 20,* 147-152.

Tressoldi, P.E., Vio C., Lorusso, M.L., Facoetti A., and Iozzino R., (2003). Confronto di efficacia ed efficienza tra trattamenti per migliorare la lettura in soggetti dislessici. *Psicologia Clinica dello Sviluppo, VII, 3,* 481-493.

Vidnyanszky, Z., and Sohn, W. (2005).Learning to suppress task-irrelevant visual stimuli with attention. *Vision Research, 45,* 677-685.

Wechsler, D. (1986). *Scala di Intelligenza Wechsler per Bambini- Riveduta.* Firenze: Organizzazioni Speciali.

Wise, B.W., and Olson, R.K. (1991). Remediating reading disabilities. In J.E. Obrzut and G.W. Hynd (Eds.), *Neuropsychological foundations of learning disabilities.* New York: Academic Press. pp. 631-658.

INDEX

W

weakness, 113

Y

young adults, ix, 79, 82